Easy Peas-y

ISBN 97986

by Emilia

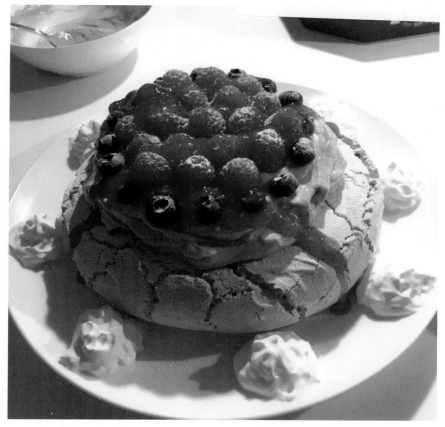

Can you believe that this contains absolutely no animal products or gluten?!

To put it simply, I genuinely think that the food in this cookbook is delicious, nutritious, and easy to make. So, I don't really see the point in eating food that is more expensive, bad for the environment and harmful to animals, when you could just cook the food in this book.

It is as easy peas-y as that.

Foreword

You may ask, how I came to take this life-changing route? Well, it all started when my Dad bought me the Leon 'FAST VEGAN' cookbook for Christmas, which really inspired me. For my family, I think the seed was sown after I came home for the holidays and cooked tasty vegetarian/vegan dishes for them every day. But it was only after they watched a documentary about plant-based diets, that I got a text from my mum that said, 'Right, we are going plant-based today.' I remember her sending me a pic of her first vegan dinner - beans on toast, but with peanut butter in place of dairy butter!

What a lot of fun we had coming our way, and hopefully you will have the same fun too.

This is not just a diet, this is a lifestyle change, but if you stick with it, 6 months down the line you will really see the difference in yourself, in the way you think, look and feel. Small steps give big changes. It's like exercise; don't say, 'I can't do that,' just take small steps and add in a little every day. Before you know it, you will be feeling on top of the world. Make these into habits of a lifetime and you will never look back.

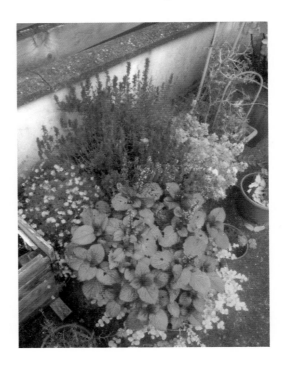

My mum's first cup of tea without good old cows' milk was dreadful. She really regretted saying that she would go plant-based. But after a few days, she grew to like the taste of tea with oat milk, and we all noticed that she no longer made those 'oooh, argh, my joints are stiff' kind of noises when she got up. Added to this, her cholesterol was previously on the high side, but 6 months down the line her bad cholesterol is now low. My dad has tried to lose weight his whole life, but since going plant-based, he's found he's been able to eat plenty of delicious food but still get into the shape he wants - no more calorie counting for him. The best part of all, unlike other diets, this lifestyle is sustainable. My older brother loves how easy it is to cook without meat or dairy - no having to worry about accidentally getting food poisoning from undercooked chicken, or out of date milk! My younger brother loves learning about the environmental impacts of our actions and trying to improve his own carbon footprint. For me, I love the challenge of trying to make dishes without just relying on meat to make them tasty. In addition, there is very little freezer space in my house at uni, so I wanted a diet that involved lots of tinned and dried food (like beans and lentils).

We are firm believers in enriching the world we live in, so we started growing our own edible flowers, herbs, fruit and vegetables. We are very fortunate to have a little garden, but you should try it even if you don't. You don't need much space - fresh basil picked off your windowsill; mint in little pots outside your door growing so wild that you can't eat enough of it; marjoram and the joy you will get when it flowers, attracting masses of bees busily buzzing around - to think they grew from the sprinkling of a little seed way back in May. Have you ever tried to grow a courgette? If not, why not? You will be so surprised - from one little plant you will get bundles of courgettes so fresh and tasty. Lettuce is another - no more soggy lettuce in a plastic bag. Look into it... you may just be shocked at what you can achieve with a few small pots on a windowsill. (On the next page is basil and mint grown on my lovely friend Nash's windowsill).

This brings me to plastic - we try to buy all our fresh fruit and vegetables from our local market. We can walk or cycle there and they deliver, plus we often get a good deal with items thrown in if we go at the end of the day. But the best bit is that there is barely any plastic used. When I'm at university I go to the local market for my fruit and veg and they give a 25% discount for students!!! In addition, dairy free milk comes in Tetra Pak cartons which have the lowest environmental impact when recycling, much better than plastic dairy milk bottles.

Another way to reduce plastic is to sprout your own beans or seeds, such as bean sprouts or Nigella seeds. These can add a lot of flavour to dishes and serve as a great way to add extra nutrients and minerals too.

Then there is the money saved. Just think - a tub of hummus in a single-use plastic pot may cost you £1 say, but if you make the delicious homemade variety (pg 156), it will taste better, use no plastic, cost about a quarter of the price AND it won't cost the Earth.

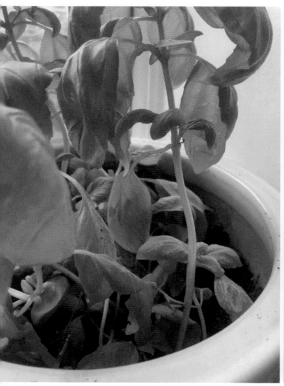
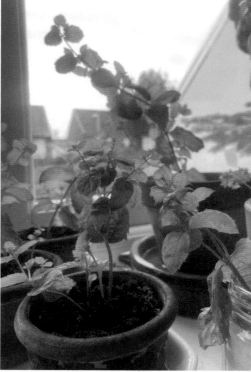

We could also get to the nitty gritty. The Amazon Rainforest is being destroyed every day for soya and palm oil production (where at least 80% of soya goes to cattle feed alone[1]); the overuse of antibiotics in cattle farms, resulting in antibiotic resistant superbugs[2]; the mistreatment and slaughter of animals; overfishing, which causes damage to marine ecosystems; the burning of fossil fuels; the significant environmental impact of the textile and clothing fast fashion industry[3]; the overuse of preservatives and food processing pre-packaged plastic meals[4] - this is all costing you and the Earth.

We don't need to live like this - you can make the change; think...

- Do I need to take the car; get a rucksack and perhaps walk or cycle?
- Shop at your local market and buy what's in season - it's fun to find out *and* saves you money.
- Make your own breakfast cereal.
- Drink hemp/oat milk (the best milks for the environment).
- Buy organic when you can.
- Eat a variety of foods.
- Steer clear of plastic-wrapped biscuits that have used unsustainable palm oil - make your own.
- Grow your own - try just one of these: herbs, sprouted beans, fruit or vegetables.
- When you can Reduce, Reuse, Recycle and buy local.
- Buy in bulk, it saves you money and reduces plastic. If you struggle to buy in bulk, save up the money you would've spent on chicken or beef and use that. I splashed out on a big bag of rice at uni and it lasted me the whole year (even though one of my housemates dropped it on the floor and split the bag open on the first day haha).

[1] https://globalforestatlas.yale.edu/amazon/land-use/soy
[2] https://www.ncbi.nlm.nih.gov/pmc/articles/PMC4638249/
[3] https://www.europarl.europa.eu/RegData/etudes/BRIE/2019/633143/EPRS_BRI(2019)633143_EN.pdf
[4] https://citeseerx.ist.psu.edu/viewdoc/download?doi=10.1.1.735.3047&rep=rep1&type=pdf

A final note before we begin -

I haven't put timings into making most recipes because often it just depends how quickly you can chop!

However, the SIMPLE SUPPER dishes are slightly different -

- I've put codes in to help you navigate timings 🕐, if it's reheatable Ⓗ or if it's freezable ❄.
- I've priced the Tomato and Chorizo Jambalaya (pg 105) and Chilli Sin Carne (pg 114) as examples of how little a delicious and nutritious dinner can cost you
- You could chop and change the ingredients to suit your needs, for example you could:
  - remove the garlic and ginger
  - If you don't have a variety of herbs, just use dried 'mixed herbs'
  - swap, let's say, the courgettes for another vegetable depending what you like or have in
  - play around with the recipe to see what suits you, but follow the vegetable cooking time instructions (pg 49).

All the recipes in this book are kind to you, your pocket, animals and the planet -

what more could you want?

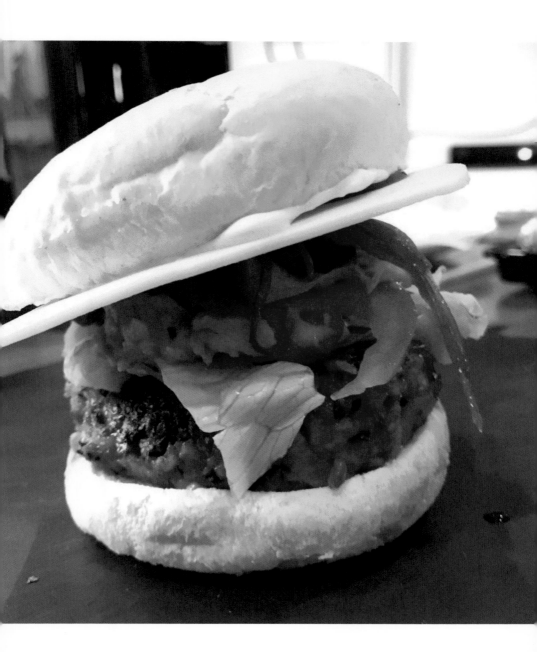

DISCLAIMER:

If you have any medical conditions or need a specific diet, then seek a professional for advice before following this lifestyle.

Table of Contents

START 12

SETUP.. 14

Cutting an Onion 14

Cutting a Pepper 16

Preparing an Avocado 18

Preparing Cauliflower 19

Preparing Garlic 20

Squeezing Firm Tofu.. 22

How to get the most juice out of a lemon/lime 23

Lentils... 24

Sprouting Beans and Seeds 26

Egg Replacements 27

How to cook your grains 28

SUNRISE 32

Su's Granola (inspired by a good friend) 32

Porridge 34

Grandad Pete's Breakfast Muffins 36

Scrambled Tofu on Toast 37

Big Boy's Breakfast 38

SALADS 40

Mango and Cabbage Salad... 40

Coleslaw.. 40

Ged's Potato Salad 41

Kat's Coleslaw 41

Mediterranean Couscous/Quinoa Salad 42

Classic Russell Salad.. 43

Falafel Salad... 44

Goat's Cheese Salad.. 46

SOUPS 47

Hearty Barley Broth 47

Table of cooking times for vegetables.....................49

Seb's Ramen...50

Mum's Tomato Soup.......................................52

SIMPLE SUPPERS..54

'Tuna' Pasta 🖐 Ⓗ...55

Loaded Pesto Pasta 🖐🖐 Ⓗ............................56

Cashew and Spinach Pasta 🖐🖐 Ⓗ 58

Spaghetti Bolognese 🖐🖐 Ⓗ ❄.....................60

Lasagne using Leftover Bolognese Sauce 🖐🖐 Ⓗ ❄ 62

Spinach and Sausage Penne 🖐 Ⓗ...................64

Spaghetti Carbonara 🖐🖐 Ⓗ..........................66

Aitken Mac 'no' Cheese 🖐🖐 Ⓗ......................68

Jacket Potato Fillings 🖐..71

Mushroom Tagliatelle 🖐 Ⓗ............................74

Dad's Roast Mushroom and Vegetable Pie 🖐🖐 Ⓗ...........76

Shepherd's Pie 🖐🖐🖐 78

Leek and Mushroom Pie 🖐🖐 Ⓗ.....................81

Thai Curry 🖐🖐 Ⓗ...84

Fried Rice 🖐..86

Su's Stir Fry 🖐🖐 Ⓗ......................................88

Satay Skewers 🖐🖐 Ⓗ...................................91

Pad Thai 🖐 Ⓗ...94

Spiced Jackfruit and Quinoa Plate 🖐🖐.............97

Sweet Potato Tagine 🖐 Ⓗ ❄ 100

Paella 🖐🖐 Ⓗ..102

Tomato and Chorizo Jambalaya 🖐 Ⓗ............105

Sweet Potato Curry 🖐 Ⓗ ❄ 108

9

Roasted Vegetable Korma 🤚🤚 Ⓗ ❄ 110

Butter Tofu 🤚 Ⓗ ❄ 112

Chilli sin Carne 🤚 Ⓗ ❄ 114

Nachos 🤚 117

Theo's Fruity Curry 🤚 Ⓗ ❄ 118

SAUCES 120

Aubergine Pasta Sauce 120

Stringy Cheese Sauce 120

Classic Tomato Sauce 121

Raspberry Coulis 121

Balsamic Glaze 122

Mint Yoghurt Dressing 122

Tahini Dressing 122

Salad Dressing 123

Silken Tofu Sour Cream 123

SATURDAYS AND SUNDAYS 124

Sushi with Watermelon 'Tuna' 124

Pizzas 130

Sweet and Sour Tofu 134

Foley Bean Burger 137

SIDES 140

Roasted Sweet Potatoes 140

Dad's Dal 142

Auntie Shoba's Dal 145

My Take on Bruschetta 146

Simple Salsa 147

Guacamole 147

Minted Peas 148

Caramelised Red Onion 148

Easy Peasy Edamames 149

Toasted Cashews 149

Tempeh.. 150

Crispy Tofu Pieces 152

Miso Glazed Aubergines 154

Cauliflower Cheese 155

SNACKS... 156

Hummus 156

Tapenade 158

Flapjack with an Edge 159

Roasted Chickpeas 162

Toasties... 163

Nutty Banana Bread 164

SWEETS 166

Grandad Pete's Lemon Drizzle Cake 166

Chocolate Crispy Cakes 168

Seb's Macarons 169

Dorset Apple Cake 172

Peppermint Chocolate Heart... 174

Coconut Chia Pudding.. 176

Gluten Free Brownie 176

Raspberry Pavlova.. 178

Banoffee Pie 181

Sorbets.. 184

Easy Ice Cream... 186

Equipment.. 188

Index 190

Definitions of Unfamiliar Ingredients........................... 191

A FINAL WORD.. 194

START - *Where to start?*

I suggest that you do an initial basic shop for all the necessities... These are the go-to staples to help you on your way to being plant-based and surviving that first week. Don't waste and throw out any old stuff you may have, use it up, but then start shopping the new way.

- Oat/hemp milk - it won't go off so buy plenty.
- 2 packs of 'Pure dairy-free spread' one for cooking and one for spreading - I believe this brand is the most environmentally friendly that I can find (they use sustainably sourced palm oil).
- Sunflower oil for cooking.
- Coconut oil.
- A loaf of bread - sourdough and ciabatta don't contain soy or palm oil, if you have allergies you may require gluten-free like Warburtons sourdough in a brown bag - you will have to decide this. We have had a bread machine for all my life - this has saved us a fortune in money and on the plastic bags.
- Peanut butter - Meridian's variety does not use palm oil, contains no sugar, and is extremely tasty. Buy the largest one you can save on plastic waste.
- Marmite - it does contain barley, wheat, oats, rye and celery in case you are intolerant, otherwise it is full of vitamin B and great for you. Buy the largest pot you can.
- Baked beans.
- A great big bag of oats in a cardboard box or paper bag.
- A jar of local honey.
- Locally grown jam.
- Bags of seeds, nuts and dried fruit - if you go to your market you may be able to buy them loose in brown bags (I'd say I use cashews, sunflower seeds and flax seeds the most).
- Flour - when I'm at Mum's we have to have gluten-free, but a bag of plain, self-raising and cornflour will do.
- Soy sauce - Kikkoman has the fewest ingredients (additives and preservatives) although I try to find sauce using GM soy as it means less pesticides used. Get a gluten free one if need be.
- Worcester sauce is an easy item to use to replace flavour that would've otherwise come from meat, however it often contains a small amount of anchovies (a fish), so I like to use Chippa Worcester Sauce from Asda, which is gluten free, anchovy free and preservative free.
- Apple cider vinegar.

- Stock cubes: Marmite is the best if you aren't gluten intolerant; Knorr is good because they are gluten free but do use a little palm oil; Marigold Bouillon vegan is good, but a little more pricey.
- Salt, pepper, herbs and spices (paprika and smoked paprika are really good for adding a meaty taste, garam masala is a really good all-rounder and Italian seasoning is good for pasta dishes).
- Quinoa (an amazing side that is actually a seed, so full of protein).
- Pasta, rice and noodles - the largest bags you can find.
- Chickpeas, dried/tins of beans (dried beans are a really good way of saving money; however, I wouldn't advise getting dried kidney beans as they have to be soaked for a minimum of 8 hours).
- Dried lentils.
- Hemp hearts (these amazing little seeds are actually a complete protein, like meat, and are perfect for sprinkling on any meal)
- Tins of tomatoes (unless it's summer and you can buy loads of fresh ones locally grown).
- Coconut milk.
- Oat biscuits.
- Vegan cheese.
- Hummus, good for a snack when you're unsure what to eat, have with pitta bread, carrots or celery.
- Frozen peas, chips, edamame beans and spinach.
- Locally grown fruit and vegetables from your market.
- Multivitamin from The Vegan Society to ensure that you are getting enough vitamin B12 & iodine.

SETUP - *a few handy things to know.*

Cutting an Onion

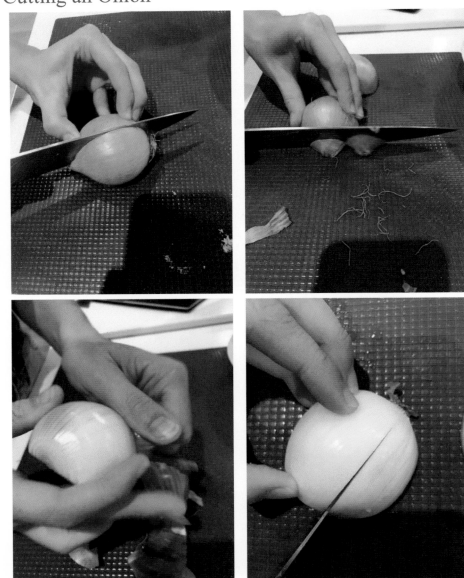

For Finely Diced

Step 1: Cut the onion in half lengthways.

Step 2: Cut the non- 'hairy' ends off. I don't know if it's true, but my older brother told me that the 'hairy' bit is where the chemical that makes you cry comes from, so if you leave chopping that until the very end your eyes won't water as much.

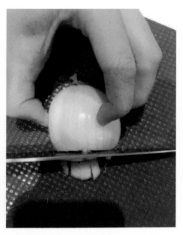

Step 3: Peel off the skin.

Step 4: Make incisions along the onion, up to the 'hairy' bit. By not cutting all the way off, it makes the next part easier.

Step 5: Cut perpendicular to the incisions we just made, this results in quick, uniform, finely diced pieces.

Step 6 (not pictured): When it gets awkward to cut, turn the onion so that the 'hairy' part is facing up then just cut around it.

If you want it even more finely diced, add in a step 4.5 where you make incisions parallel to the chopping board.

For Crescent Moons

For Rings

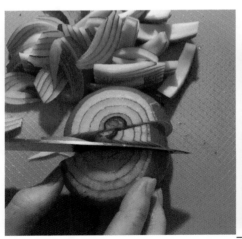

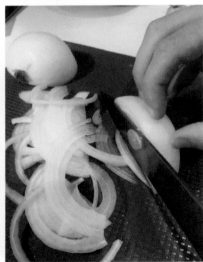

Cutting a Pepper

This method actually came to me in a dream, I've never met anyone else who does it like this (although I'm sure there will be someone somewhere), but I think it is by far the best method.

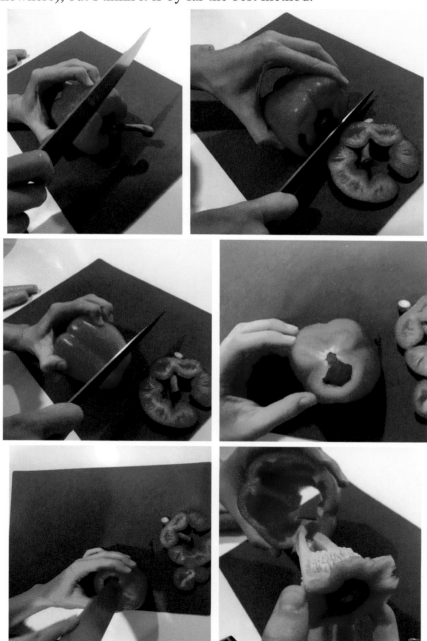

Step 1: Cut the top off the pepper (fairly close to the end so that the base of the stalk remains attached to the core ideally).

Step 2: Cut the bottom off the pepper, now you should be able to see the core and see that it attaches to the rest of the pepper with pale strands.

Step 3: Using your knife (in the wider opening) cut these strands and the core will come out perfectly intact, no seed clean-up required.

Step 4: Put the core and the green stem in the food waste bin/compost bin and cut all the remaining pepper however you would like.

For Slices

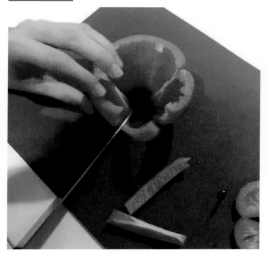

For Chunks

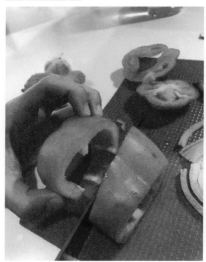
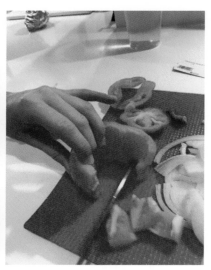

Preparing an Avocado

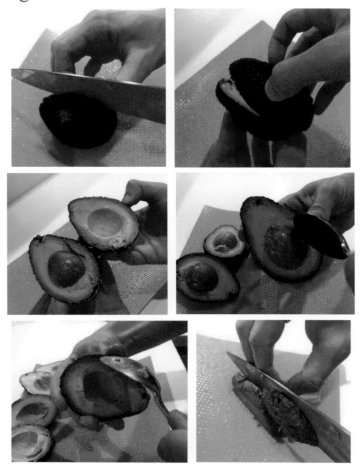

Step 1: Cut the avocado in half lengthways, pivoting the knife around the stone in the middle.

Step 2: Twist the top and the bottom of the avocado until both halves come apart.

Step 3: Lever the stone out with a spoon (some people use a knife and impale the stone with it, but I think this works just as well and is far less stressful).

Step 4: Scoop out the flesh (eurgh) with the spoon.

Step 5: Cut into slices.

Preparing Cauliflower

Step 1: Cut the leaves off the bottom.

Step 2: Make a cross in the bottom of the stalk - this will enable the stalk and florets to cook for the same amount of time.

Step 3: Place the cauliflower stalk side down in a large Pyrex bowl with a tablespoon of water, cover and microwave for 8 minutes until slightly soft or to your liking.

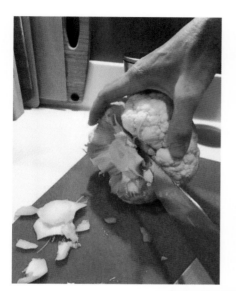
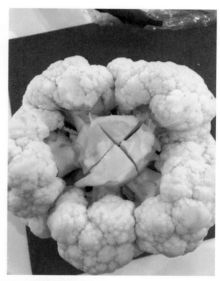

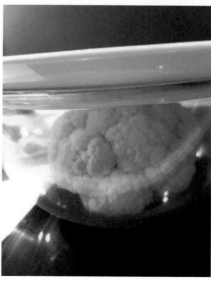

Preparing Garlic

If you like the taste of garlic, crush it (with a garlic crusher) to bring out a stronger flavour than chopping. The idea is that the more garlic cells you break, the more alliinase is converted into allicin (which is the thing that gives the smell of fresh garlic), therefore a stronger garlic flavour.

If you're using garlic raw, but want a slightly milder taste, the key thing is to let the chopped/crushed garlic sit for about 10 minutes before you use it in your recipe. This is because allicin is unstable and breaks down into other compounds, reducing the potency. Alternatively, squeeze some lemon/lime juice on your garlic as this denatures the alliinase in a similar way to cooking.

If you aren't a huge fan of garlic in general (like my great Auntie Valerie), but still want to include it in a dish, roast it whole as this means that no garlic cells have been broken, resulting in a sweet and mild taste.

Garlic should be stored in a warm, dry place i.e. not in the fridge.

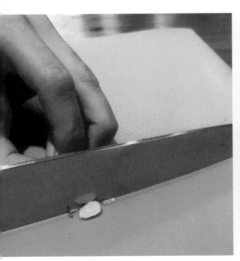
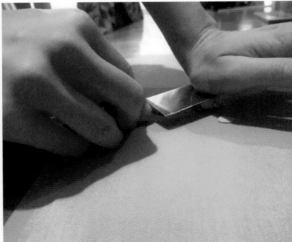

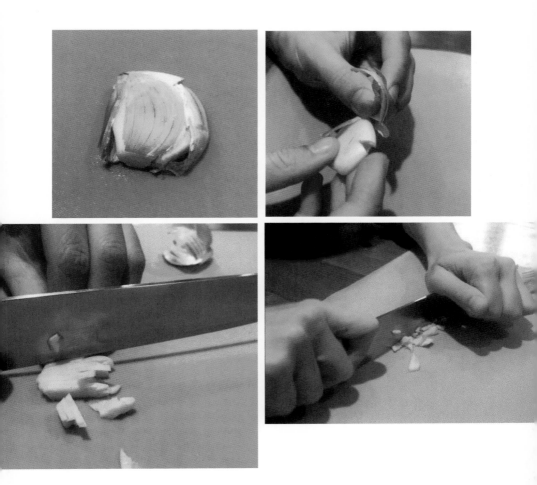

Step 1: Cut off the hard end of the garlic clove.

Step 2: Using the heel of your hand on the flat of the knife, push down on the garlic until you hear a crack.

Step 3: The skin should come off the clove very easily now, so hopefully your fingers won't end up smelling of garlic.

Step 4: Finely slice the garlic.

Step 5: Move the knife up and down repeatedly over the clove, moving your dominant hand forward and backward, while keeping the end of the knife in the same position with your non-dominant hand (it is essentially acting as a pivot).

Squeezing Firm Tofu

This is a very important step if you want your tofu to be crispy and hold its shape as there is a lot of liquid stored inside that results in crumblier tofu. If you are using the tofu in scrambled tofu or just in a saucy dish, this step is optional.

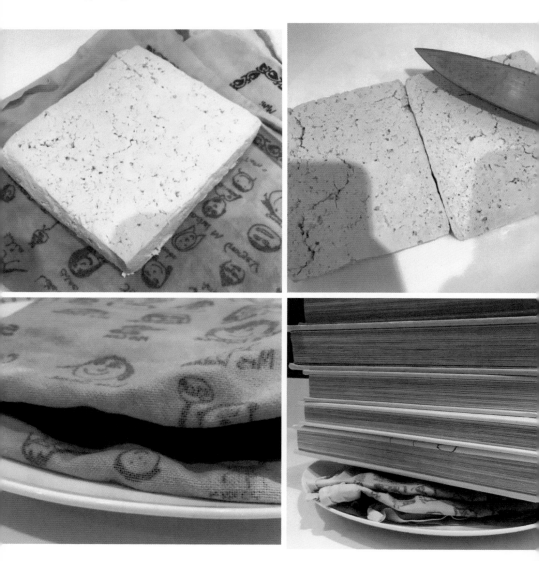

Step 1: Take the firm tofu out of the water in the packet and gently squeeze it in your hands to remove some liquid.

Step 2: Cut the tofu in half widthways. Increasing the surface area helps to squeeze out a lot more water, but only do it if you don't need big chunks of tofu in your final recipe.

Step 3: Wrap the tofu in kitchen roll/a clean tea towel.

Step 4: Place something heavy on top, like lots of cookbooks or tins of beans, and leave for 10-20 minutes. This may seem like a lot of time, but it requires far less forethought than defrosting beef/chicken.

Check on your tofu halfway, if the kitchen roll is saturated with water, replace with some dry sheets and continue to press.

You can buy a 'tofu press' online if you want but we think this method works fine.

Alternatively, you can freeze the tofu while still in the packaging (takes about 4 hours), then boil for 15 minutes to defrost (flipping halfway). You can then use the tofu as usual (for example in my crispy tofu pieces recipe on pg 153), without having to squeeze out the water.

How to get the most juice out of a lemon/lime

1. Roll it under the heel of your hand to crush the pulp, making more juice come out when you squeeze it.
2. Microwave for 15 seconds to ripen.
3. If you're using a lime, just stick your thumbs in and squeeze that way as limes have no seeds!

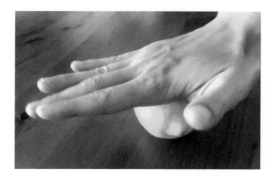

Lentils

I typically use about 50g lentils per person which is ¼ mug for me.

Lentils are amazing because they are really nutritious and really cheap if you buy them dry. They are also blank slates, so they absorb all the flavour of the sauce they're in. In our house, we predominantly work with 2 different coloured lentils, brown (or puy if we can't get brown) and red.

Brown/Puy

I like to use these lentils in the place of minced beef/minced lamb etc and in salads. They hold their shape really well (unlike red lentils), no matter how you cook them, so they are really great if you're new to the world of lentils. They are quite small in size but bulk up a lot when cooked. If you are not keen on giving up meat completely, these can still be a great part of your diet if you add them to chillies/spag bols etc as they pass by unnoticed, while bulking up your meal, therefore saving money.

Red

These are good in soups and dals as they break up a little bit, thickening the sauce and adding some extra nutrients. Red lentils also have the shortest cooking time so if you're in a rush, a red lentil dish is the way to go. Alternatively, buying pre-cooked lentils works well too.

Table of cooking times for dried lentils:

Brown/Green: Boil for 35-45 minutes with plenty of water

Puy: Simmer for 15-25 minutes with plenty of water

Red: Add to sauce boil for 10 minutes and simmer for 7-
                       15 minutes

Top Tips:

Always rinse your lentils thoroughly before use, removing any shrivelled lentils.

The table above is for boiling in *water* (for brown, green and puy), I would advise cooking in the sauce you want them in for extra flavour, however, this will result in varying cooking times so make sure that the lentils are soft (can be crushed between your fingers) before you eat them.

Adding salt increases the cooking time and makes the lentils firmer, so try to add any salt at the end of the cooking process.

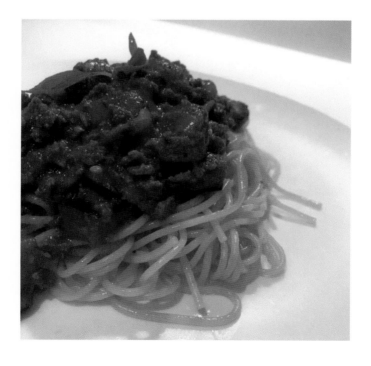

Sprouting Beans and Seeds

Sprouting beans and pulses are excellent for adding packs of nutrition to your diet and will add bags of flavour and texture to your meal. The process of sprouting increases the nutritional value of protein, folate, magnesium, phosphorus, vitamin C and K.

It is easy to do, economical, and saves a lot of plastic compared to buying them from the shops.

The basic principles are: Soak, usually overnight, Rinse, Drain, Air circulation, Store and Cleanliness.

Use the whole sprouted bean or seed raw or quickly stir fried.

Don't use seeds that have been chemically treated. However, other than that, they don't need to be especially for sprouting, just a bag of in-date dried beans or seeds will do.

Seeds should not be left to sprout so long that rootlets appear as they can become tough.

Not all sprouting seeds and beans are edible.

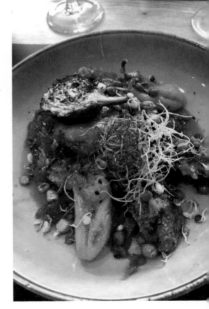

All you need is a jar and a little time... check out YouTube for more instructions.

Seed	Uses	Rinsing	Ready after
Fenugreek	Salads, soups, curries	2-3 times a day	4-7 days
Lentils whole	Salads and soups	2-3 times a day	3-4 days
Mung beans	Stir fries and salads	3 times daily	4-5 days
Radish sprouts	Salads, sandwiches	2-3 times daily	3-4 days when sprouts visible
Sesame	Salads	3-4 times a day	3-4 days when sprouts visible

Egg Replacements

1 egg = 1 tbsp of ground flax seeds + 3 tbsp of water, then leave to sit

1 egg = 1 tbsp chia seeds, finely ground + 3 tbsp water, then leave to sit

1 egg = 3 tbsp chickpeas water (after the can has been shaken)

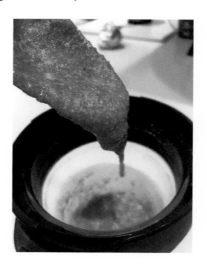

How to cook your grains

My main advice for this whole section is do everything (except couscous) by volume i.e. always measure your water and grains in a mug/jug. For me **1 mug water = 280g.**

Pasta

Pasta is very easy and very tasty; the cooking time is slightly different for gluten free pasta (see the instructions on the packet) but the same principles apply.

Allow roughly 80g dry pasta per person.

Boil plenty of water in the kettle and put the pasta into a large pan.

Add the water to the pasta and bring to the boil. If you have a stove that isn't very efficient, I advise adding the pasta once the water is boiling so that you don't get soggy pasta.

Season the water generously with salt (it should taste like the sea) and cook for 8-10 minutes, depending on the type of pasta and how al dente (firm) you like it.

For me **1 mug pasta = 80g.**

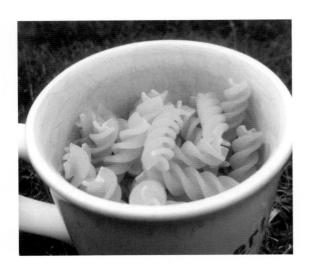

Rice

My favourite rice is basmati, it is really tasty and really easy to cook. If you follow my instructions, not only will you fall in love with basmati too, you will also save lots of money because you can buy 10kg bags of basmati for £12, that means it's 9p per portion!

Allow about 75-80g dry rice per person, it is best to have a standard mug where you know how much rice it holds (for me **1 mug of rice = 200g**).

Pour your rice into a saucepan (beware, rice expands a lot so don't use a really small pan) and add some water.

Swish the rice around with your hand for a few minutes until the water is cloudy with starch, then empty the rice into a sieve and give it a rinse with running water.

Pour the rice into a pan and heat on a low heat, with a little oil, while you measure the water to toast the grains a little **OPTIONAL**.

Measure out double the amount of water to rice BY VOLUME (i.e. if you used ½ a mug of rice, do 1 mug of water; if you used 2 mugs of rice, do 4 mugs of water) and pour the water into the pan.

Add about ½ tsp salt per person to the water, stir **once** and then bring to a boil. Rice is quite fragile so if you stir it lots, you will break the grains, releasing more starch which will make your rice mushy.

As soon as the rice has come to the boil, reduce the heat to low and put the lid on.

Cook for 10-15 minutes until the rice is soft through then take off the heat.

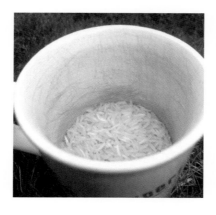

Quinoa

Fun fact, quinoa is actually not a grain, it's a seed! Which means that not only is it gluten free, it is also full of protein. I used to really dislike quinoa because of how we cooked it, but I found a recipe from wendypolisi.com (basically the Queen of Quinoa) and now I actually really like quinoa.

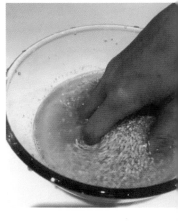

Allow roughly 40g dry quinoa per person, that is ⅕th of a mug for me. For me **1 mug of quinoa = 210g**.

Rinse the quinoa thoroughly, either under running water or in a bowl, this helps to stop the quinoa sticking together when cooked and also helps to make it less bitter.

While you're rinsing, feel free to fry some garlic/onions/peppers etc in the quinoa pan to make it even more full of flavour.

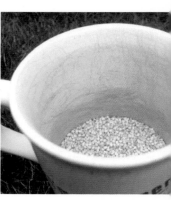

Drain and place in a medium size pan and dry fry to toast the seed to bring out the flavour.

Add water in the ratio of 1:1.25 (mugs of quinoa to mugs of water) with 1 stock cube.

i.e. for a family of 5, you do 1 mug of quinoa, 1.25 mugs of water. I would recommend cooking quinoa in bulk as it is a lot easier to do the right amount of water and it stores really well, but if you are doing a small amount, just do the same amount of quinoa to water and then add a dash more water.

Bring to the boil and then reduce to a low heat.

Cook for 30-35 minutes with the lid on, then take off the heat and leave to stand for another 5 minutes.

Add a drizzle of extra virgin olive oil/a knob of vegan butter and fluff up the quinoa with a fork.

Couscous

We don't eat couscous very much anymore because it isn't suitable for people who are gluten intolerant, however, for people who aren't gluten intolerant it is the easiest grain to cook in my opinion.

If you're putting lots of extras with the couscous, i.e. chopped cherry tomatoes, nuts, seeds etc, allow roughly 50g dry couscous per person.

If you're having it plain as a side, allow 70g dry couscous per person. For me, **1 mug of couscous = 230g**.

Pour the couscous into a large bowl, with a stock cube and place on the scales.

Boil the kettle with plenty of water.

Pour [1.5x the amount of couscous] grams of water into the large bowl and mix to ensure that the stock cube has dissolved.

I.e. if you're doing 1 plain portion of couscous, you should use 1.5 x 70 = 105g of water, if you're doing 3 loaded portions, use 1.5 x 150 = 225g water. If you don't have scales, a measuring jug works just as well as 1g of water = 1ml of water.

Then cover the bowl with a plate or a lid and leave the couscous to stand for 5 minutes or until the couscous is completely soft.

Then take the lid off, drizzle in a little extra virgin olive oil and fluff up the couscous with a fork.

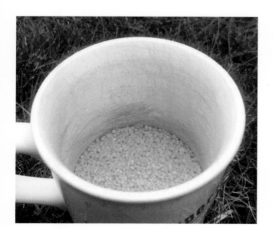

SUNRISE - *Breakfast is reportedly the best meal of the day, once you have tried our homemade granola you will never look back.*

Su's Granola (inspired by a good friend)
Roughly 20 portions

This is a mix and match recipe; you can vary the ingredients as to what you have in the cupboard. For example, if you don't have apricots but you have some dried blueberries - then hey - who are we to disagree!

10 mins to put together
40 mins cook

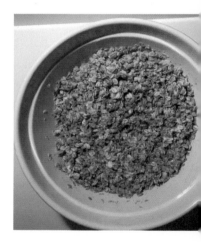

Ingredients
250ml sunflower oil

2 tbsp of coconut oil

100ml honey

1 tsp of each: cinnamon and mixed spices

650g jumbo oats

¾ tsp salt

150g of dried apricots, washed and chopped

50g of desiccated coconut

50g of sesame seeds

50g of chia seeds

50g of sunflower seeds

50g of pumpkin seeds

(optional: 50g dry quinoa and 50g hemp hearts, for extra protein)

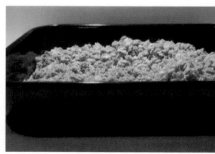

80g of dried cranberries

50g of hazelnuts

50g of walnuts

50g brazil nuts

50gs pecan nuts

20g macadamia nuts

50g of almonds

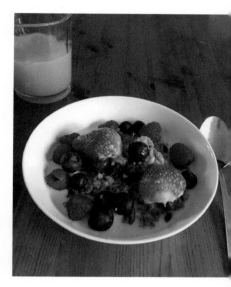

Method

Place into a large microwaveable bowl:

- 250ml sunflower oil
- 2 tbsp of coconut oil,
- A large pour of honey (roughly 100ml),

Melt on LOW power setting/heat in the microwave, until all melted.

Preheat the oven to around 110°C/130°C fan.

Stir the oil and honey mix, then add the salt, ground cinnamon and mixed spices.

Pour in the jumbo oats.

Stir well, making sure all the oats are coated in this mixture.

Place into a clean large baking tray (the one we use is 32 x 26 x 7cm), I cover the tray with tin foil so that no old bits of pizza from the oven get into my cereal!

Cook for 30 mins. Stir once during cooking.

After 30 mins, add as many seeds, nuts or dried fruit as you fancy. I break up the walnuts and brazil nuts before adding to the mixture and chop the washed dried apricots.

Place back in the oven for 10 mins to release the flavour of the nuts and seeds. The Granola should look golden.

Store on an airtight container... You will have eaten it before it goes off! Enjoy with vegan yoghurt (we like Alpro) or oat milk, and fresh fruit.

Porridge

I like to make my porridge in the ratio **1:2, fine oats : non-dairy milk** (by volume) and then pop it in the microwave for around 2 minutes at 1000W. I have a favourite mug and half of that mug is 1 serving for me (ie, half a mug of oats, mixed with 1 mug of milk), so that I don't have to weigh it out every day. This is around 50g of oats for one portion, but it takes a few tries to find what's perfect for you.

If you make it for more people, do it in a big bowl and multiply 2 minutes by 1.5 for every extra portion, i.e. for 3 people it will take 2x1.5x1.5 = 4.5 mins.

I think that using fine oats helps to make a really creamy porridge with no effort. I also think that using milk is 100000x better than using water because it only costs a little more but results in much creamier porridge and there are also added vitamins in dairy-free milk, which help contribute to a healthy diet. If you don't have any milk, adding ½ tsp of salt per person does help to make a creamier porridge in a pinch.

Alternatively, quinoa can be used instead of oats, in the ratio 1:3, quinoa:non-dairy milk, however, that is best done on the hob, simmered for 15-20 minutes.

Toppings
- Honey/agave nectar (for the strict vegans) - it's a classic for a reason.
- Cinnamon and sliced banana - this is best if you put the banana in as soon as the porridge comes out of the microwave which results in the scrummiest caramelised banana flavour.
- A spoonful of your favourite jam (I always go for raspberry).
- A spoonful of palm oil-free crunchy peanut butter for a nice change in texture.
- A sprinkle of mixed seeds/chopped nuts on top for those extra vitamins and good fats.
- A dollop of dairy free creme fraiche or yoghurt for a fresh tang.
- Assorted fruit, it is most cost effective to buy the fruit that is in season, so I've included a table below to help you know what to get at what times of year.

Spring (March - June)	Strawberries, raspberries, blueberries
Summer (June- September)	Blackberries, apples
Autumn (September - December)	Pears
Winter (December - March)	Bananas, tinned/frozen fruit

For a bit of a funky twist, try making your porridge with coconut milk (out of a carton, not a tin) and serve it with pineapple for a piña colada vibe (see below).

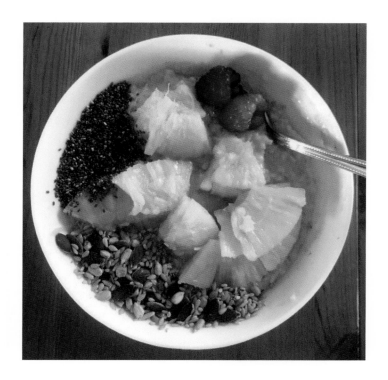

Grandad Pete's Breakfast Muffins

Makes about 12

You will need a muffin tray.

These are really tasty, filling and high in fibre so make a good weekend breakfast. I like to batch make them, freeze them, and then take two out, defrost them, slice them in half, grill them and spread some vegan butter on top. This recipe also does not need to be very precise, so I like to pick a mug (with a volume of around 240ml if you want to be precise) and use that in place of a scale. If you use a smaller mug, use slightly less 'egg'.

Ingredients

3 flax 'eggs'

1 mug of soft light brown sugar

½ mug of vegetable oil

2 mugs non-dairy milk (I think oat milk works well here)

2½ mugs plain flour (can use gf)

2½ tsp bicarbonate of soda

1 tsp salt

2 mugs oat bran (there are plenty of gluten free versions available online, Amazon is a good place to start). You can also buy rice or hemp bran which I've never tried but I don't see why they wouldn't work

1 mug mixed dried fruit (I like to use sultanas)

1 mug of desiccated coconut

Method

Preheat the oven to 210°C/190°C fan.

Beat the flax eggs in a large bowl for a few minutes until they're paler and fluffier (you aren't going to get the same consistency as eggs, but you still want to try to beat air into them). Gradually add the sugar to the eggs, beating well. Slowly add the oil, continuing to beat the mixture. Separately mix the flour and the salt and then add that mixture to the eggs, along with the bicarbonate of soda, milk and bran. Mix well and stir in the fruit and the coconut. Spoon mixture into greased muffin tray, filling each hole ¾ full. Bake for 15-20 minutes, or until a skewer comes out clean.

Scrambled Tofu on Toast

Makes 2 large portions

I'm not going to lie and tell you that this is exactly the same as scrambled eggs, but it is so delicious and filling that you won't want scrambled eggs.

Ingredients

1 tbsp vegan butter (ideally, you want one that claims it tastes like butter)

2 spring onions, sliced

1 tsp black onion seeds

One block (396g in water) of firm tofu if you like your scrambled eggs quite firm OR one block (349g) of silken tofu if you like your scrambled eggs a bit softer and creamier

Splash of non-dairy milk if using firm tofu

Salt and pepper

½ tbsp nutritional yeast

Optional

Pinch of black salt (kala namak), a salt that has a high sulphur content so tastes 'eggy'

1 tsp of garlic powder to add more depth

Method

If using firm tofu, take care to squeeze out excess water before use, if unsure how, see page 22.

Heat the vegan butter in a frying pan and add the spring onions and the black onion seeds. Fry for 1-2 minutes at a medium-high to release the flavour, without making the spring onions go soggy.

Crumble your tofu of choice into the frying pan and fry on a medium heat for 5 minutes until the tofu is hot all the way through (if using garlic powder or black salt, add at this stage).

Turn the heat off, stir in the nutritional yeast and season to taste.

Top tip: nutritional yeast denatures at high heat (>100°C), so if you want the nutritional benefits, try to add it right before serving.

Enjoy with some toasted bread, slathered in vegan butter, some thin slices of tomato and a glass of orange juice.

Big Boy's Breakfast

Our 'Full English' is made up of a bunch of different components, which can be included/removed based on what we have in at the time. None of these are difficult to make, we are just including a few tips/tricks to help you make it as best a replacement for the original as possible. These are:

- **Toast with vegan butter**
- **Scrambled tofu** (pg 37)
- **Baked beans**

- **Vegan sausages**

I was going to tell you which are our favourite sausage substitutes, but talking to my family, it is clear how subjective it is, and I feel like half the fun of going plant-based is trying lots of different things to see what works for you (if you really want to know, my favourite are the Richmond Meat Free). I will say, if you want to cook your vegan sausages well, I would advise cooking them in a frying pan/oven for 5-10 minutes to defrost them, then cut them into bite size pieces, toss in a little more oil and return to the pan/oven. This makes them a lot crispier and improves the sausage eating experience greatly.

- **Mum's onion and mushroom mix**

Finely chop an onion or two, heat a little oil in a pan and sauté the onions until they are softening a little. Meanwhile slice some mushrooms pop them in with the onions, add some salt and pepper…. Cook for a further 10 - 20 minutes on a low/medium heat until the mushrooms are just how you like them. If the mixture is drying up, pop the lid on the pan then the liquid won't evaporate off.

- **Grilled tomatoes**

Cut the tomatoes in half, nick the core out, sprinkle with salt, pepper and a little sugar, leave to stand for a few minutes. Then place under a grill, or in the frying pan and cook face down for 5 minutes, flip them over and cook until soft and tasty.

- **Vegan bacon**

Quorn does a really good vegetarian bacon which contains free-range egg whites, so if you aren't too strict, these are best cooked with lots of salt on the grill. If you would prefer to avoid animal products all together, the Quorn 'smoky ham free slices' are vegan and delicious. To make them the most similar to crispy bacon, place the slices in the grill with a light wash of vegetable oil and a good seasoning of salt and grill on medium for around 5 minutes. We have tried to fry them and found that they disintegrate a little bit, so grilling is definitely the winning method. Alternatively, go on a voyage of adventure and find a vegan bacon that you like.

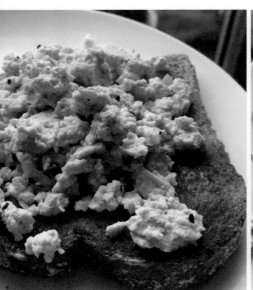 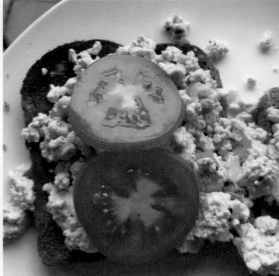

SALADS - *Not really my thing; but wait until you have tried these.*

Mango and Cabbage Salad

A large bowl

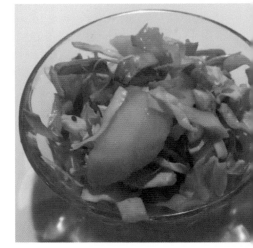

1 sweetheart cabbage finely chopped

1 mango sliced and chopped

Mix together

Serve

Store in an airtight container

Great to take on a picnic too

Coleslaw

Very large bowl

Half a white cabbage finely shredded

A few carrots medium grated

Mix with vegan mayonnaise

A dash of apple cider vinegar

Add a little salt and pepper

Great to take on a picnic or to have with a burger

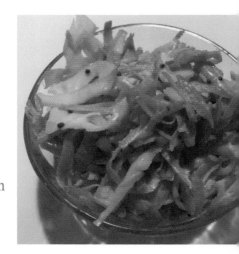

Ged's Potato Salad

Serves 6

Chop **1kg of Maris Piper potatoes** into bite-sized chunks

Boil for 20-25 mins in a large pan of salted water

Bring the potatoes to the boil from cold to ensure that they are evenly cooked through

When soft enough to stick a fork in, drain them and return to the pan

Add **4 tablespoons of extra virgin olive oil** while still hot, with **salt, pepper** and the **juice of 1 lemon**

Chop **4 spring onions** into 1cm chunks and add to the pan

Crumble in **1 block of silken tofu** (in place of egg) and add a **generous amount of vegan mayo**

Add **2 teaspoons of Dijon mustard** if you want a bit of 'bite'

Roughly chop **a handful of parsley** and stir it all to combine

Pour into a serving bowl and enjoy!

Kat's Coleslaw

Serves 12

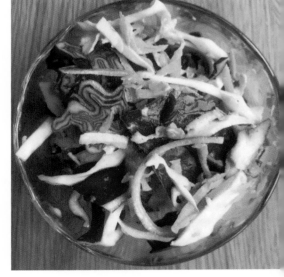

Half a red cabbage, thinly sliced

Half a white cabbage, thinly sliced

4 carrots, grated

1 apple, grated

1 red onion, thinly sliced

3 tsp Dijon mustard

2 tbsp vegan mayo (or more if you like it saucy)

Dash of apple cider vinegar

Salt and pepper

Mediterranean Couscous/Quinoa Salad

Serves 6

Ingredients

200g dry couscous or quinoa, cooked (pg 28)

2 red onions, cut into crescent moons (pg 14)

2 aubergines, cut into 2cm cubes

2 red peppers, chopped (pg 16)

2 courgettes, chopped then quartered

30 cherry tomatoes, halved

1 stock cube

½ pack/100g of vegan feta (I like the 'Violife Greek white block') - **OPTIONAL**

Oil, salt and pepper

Balsamic vinegar

A little sugar

Method

Preheat the oven to about 220°C/ 200°C fan.

Deskin and slice the red onions and put on a baking tray with a sprinkling of salt and pepper, sugar, balsamic vinegar and a drizzle of oil.

Bake the onions for 30 mins.

Wash and chop the aubergines, place on pre-oiled baking trays and season with salt and pepper.

Bake the aubergines for about 25 mins.

Wash, deseed and chop the red peppers (see pg 16 for photos on the best way to prepare a pepper).

Chop the courgettes and place the pieces onto a baking tray with the cherry tomatoes, red pepper pieces, salt, pepper and a drizzle of cooking oil.

Bake the tomatoes, peppers and courgettes for about 20 mins, or until all the vegetables are soft.

Whilst these are cooking, you can cook the quinoa/ couscous.

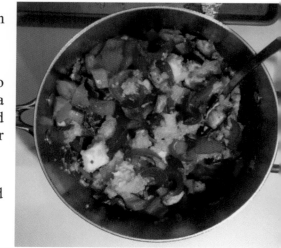

Chop the vegan goats cheese into small squares and add to the quinoa or couscous while it is still hot, add all the other ingredients and stir gently

Eat while still warm or serve cold the next day.

Store in the fridge for up to 3 days.

Great for a picnic.

Classic Russell Salad

Serves 6

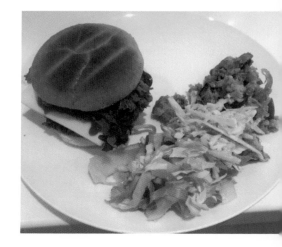

1 iceberg lettuce, cut into slices

12 cherry tomatoes, halved

Half a cucumber, thinly sliced

1 mango, cut into small cubes

2 avocados, cut into strips

2 spring onions sliced

Salt and pepper

Juice of 1 lime

Serve with dressing of your choice.

Falafel Salad

Serves 6 (makes 15 falafels)

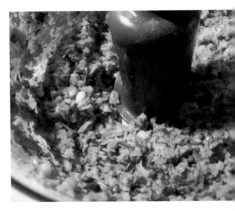

Ingredients

For the falafels

2 red onions, roughly chopped

3 cloves of garlic

1 tin of chickpeas alternatively, you could use broad beans or other white beans

1 tsp of cumin

A fresh chilli (optional)

½ tsp of paprika

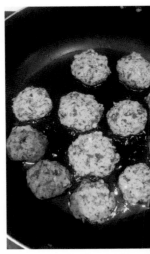

A glug of oil, ideally sesame. If you have none, use sunflower/vegetable and add a sprinkle of sesame seeds

Juice of 1 lime

Handful of fresh parsley (be generous)

Handful of fresh coriander (be generous)

1 tsp of salt

½ tsp of pepper

Plain flour (can use gf flour)

For the salad

1 Iceberg lettuce, cut into strips

2 handfuls of cherry tomatoes, halved

A handful of almonds, chopped/flaked **OPTIONAL**

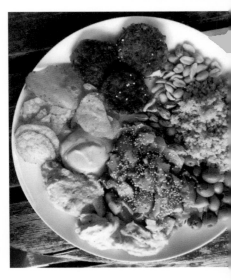

Method

Put all the falafel ingredients, except the flour, into a blender and pulse a few times to get a chunky consistency, the chickpeas should be less than ½ of their original size.

Taste and season if necessary.

Mix in a tablespoon of flour at a time until the mixture is the right consistency (you don't want it being crumbly, but you also don't want it sticking to your hands).

Pour enough oil into a frying pan so that it is around 1cm deep and heat to a medium high heat.

While the oil is heating up, roll the falafel mix into golf balls (with wet hands) and then flatten them a little to make them more into patties.

Flattening is optional, I just think that they cook better if you don't have a deep fryer

Add the falafels to the hot oil, making sure not to overcrowd the pan as this brings down the temp of the oil, and cook for 7 minutes on either side, you want them to be golden brown on the outside and hot in the middle.

Once cooked, place on a paper towel lined plate to absorb any excess oil.

While warm, toss the falafels with the sliced lettuce, tomatoes and almonds and serve with **mint yoghurt** (pg 122), **tahini dressing** (pg 122), lemon wedges or some **couscous** (pg 28).

If you'd prefer, you can bake them in the oven, on a greased baking tray, at 200°C fan for 20-30 mins, flipping halfway through.

Also, if you're feeling tired, you can buy some pre-made falafel in most supermarkets.

A blender is very handy in this recipe, but it can also be made by finely chopping the ingredients and mashing the chickpeas with a potato masher/fork.

Goat's Cheese Salad

Serves 6

The Violife 'Greek style block' is such a good replacement for feta in this salad, it gives a nice tang and melts well when warmed. We like to add roasted seasonal root vegetables, such as radishes or beetroot.

Preheat the oven to 200°C/180°C fan.

Chop **200g of root vegetables** into bite-sized pieces and place onto a baking tray with **1 tbsp of vegetable oil**, a generous sprinkle of **salt and pepper** and a **sprinkle of sugar**.

Roast for 20 minutes.

While the veg is roasting, wash **300g of rocket** and chop the **'Violife Greek white block'** (I use 100g, but my younger brother loves it so he makes this salad with the whole packet, 200g) into small chunks.

This is also a good time to make the **balsamic glaze** recipe, (pg 122).

When the roasting vegetables have 5 minutes left, put **2 handfuls of pine nuts** onto a small tray and into the oven to toast.

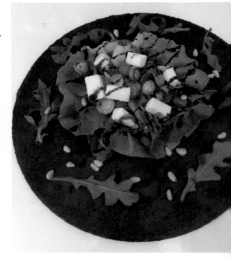

When the vegetables are soft on the inside and crispy on the outside, take them out of the oven and toss in the vegan cheese to melt it a little.

Assemble the salad by tossing together the cheese, the chopped root vegetables and the pine nuts.

Drizzle on the balsamic glaze and serve with some **apple shavings** and a nasturtium flower (if you want it to look fancy).

SOUPS - *One of my brother's favourites, especially as he received some new ramen bowls and spoons for Christmas.*

Hearty Barley Broth

Serves 6

This broth is the perfect way to use up some vegetables that are nearing the end of their life, while making a really warming and filling soup, perfect for winter evenings or days you just want a warm hug. If you are gluten intolerant, quinoa is a good replacement for the barley. This recipe calls for a big pan, but don't worry if you don't have one, just scale the recipe down accordingly.

Ingredients

This recipe is very adaptable so feel free to use other vegetables than the ones I've included, just follow the table below on how long they will need cooking.

2 onions, finely diced

5 sticks of celery, sliced into ½ cm slices

5 large garlic cloves, crushed

4cm of ginger, finely chopped

3 tsp of dried oregano

2 tsp of dried mint (or whatever dried herbs you have really)

3 vegetable stock cubes

Lots of water

¾ of a mug of pearl barley (85g) heads up, this will quadruple in size so make sure you're using a big pan OR 1 mug of quinoa (150g) if you're gluten intolerant

4 large tomatoes finely diced don't worry if you don't love tomatoes, these almost disintegrate, they're just there for the flavour

2 large carrots, sliced and quartered (to make little ½ cm high wedges)

2 sweet potatoes, cut into bite-sized cubes (2cm x 2cm)

1 swede, cut into similar sizes to the sweet potato

1 mug of frozen peas (roughly 150g)

1 mug of frozen sweetcorn (roughly 150g)

Squeeze of lemon

Method

Fry the onion and celery on a medium high heat in a deep saucepan for 5-10 minutes until the onion is translucent and they are beginning to caramelise.

Reduce the heat to medium and add the garlic, ginger and dried herbs to the onions.

If you have a gas stove, now is the perfect time to boil your water in a kettle to save time.

Once the herbs are fragrant, add about 3 litres of water to the pan with the stock cubes and stir vigorously to ensure that the stock is all dissolved.

Add the barley (if using), bring the stock to a vigorous simmer and cook for 30 minutes with the lid on.

This is a good time to prep the veg you are going to be adding, but KEEP AN EYE ON THE PAN because the barley absorbs a lot of water so you need to ensure that you are topping it up as it gets absorbed.

Add the tomatoes, carrots, sweet potatoes and swede to the broth, stirring it to ensure that nothing is sticking to the bottom of the pan and cook for another 15 minutes. *If you're using quinoa, add it now.*

By now the barley should have become soft and swollen, this means that it is time to add the peas and sweetcorn to cook for a final 5 minutes.

Add enough water to get your desired consistency and add salt, pepper and lemon juice to taste

Serve with crusty bread and vegan butter.

This stores well in an airtight container; however, you may need to top up with water as the barley will keep absorbing liquid.

I also like to keep some stock powder handy (like Bouillon) to ensure that it is still flavoursome even after adding the extra water.

Table of cooking times for vegetables
(cut into bite-sized pieces)

Hard Veg (15-20 mins)	Medium Veg (10-15 mins)	Soft Veg (2-5 mins)
Carrots	Aubergine	Spinach
Potatoes	Courgette	Beansprouts
Cauliflower	Mushrooms	Frozen peas
Parsnips	Asparagus	Mange tout

Seb's Ramen

Serves 6

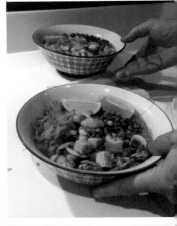

Ingredients

For the Stock

300ml water per person (1.8L overall), boiled

3 stock cubes

Start with around 6 tbsp soy sauce, but adjust to taste

1 tbsp white wine vinegar

3 tbsp apple cider vinegar

2 tbsp miso paste (any colour will do)

1 tbsp sugar

Dash sesame oil

1 tbsp curry powder

1 tin coconut milk

Salt & pepper to taste

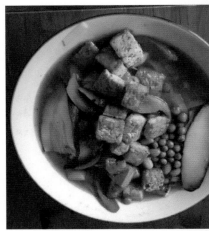

For the Crispy Tofu Pieces (like on pg 152)

1 block of firm tofu, squeezed (pg 22)

2 tbsp cornflour

2 tsp paprika

1 tsp garlic powder (optional)

1 tsp salt

Generous pinch of black pepper

Drizzle of sunflower oil

For the Topping

3 cloves garlic, chopped finely

4cm ginger, chopped finely

3 hot chillies **OPTIONAL**, sliced

500g mushrooms, sliced

Bunch of spring onions, sliced

2 mugs frozen peas (roughly 300g)

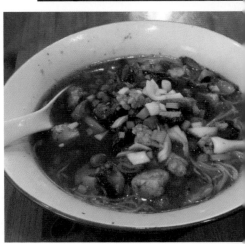

Dash soy sauce

Salt and pepper to flavour

Sprinkle of sugar

6 rice noodle nests

2 limes, cut into wedges

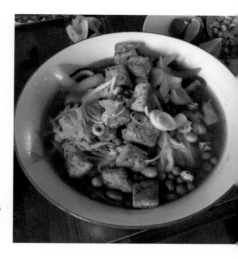

Optional Extra Topping Ideas

3 large carrots, grated

3 courgettes, thinly sliced (a peeler helps here)

Sprinkle of bean sprouts

Method

Mix together all the ingredients for the stock in a large saucepan and keep it on a very gentle simmer while you prepare the other ingredients. Make sure you taste it and adjust it to your personal taste.

Make the tofu into 'crispy tofu pieces' like on page 152 (I would recommend baking them so that they can be cooking while you prepare the other components).

Meanwhile, add the garlic, ginger and chillies to a frying pan with a dash of oil and fry on a medium heat for 5 minutes.

Add in the mushrooms and the white parts of the spring onions and cook with the lid on for around 10 minutes, until the mushrooms are soft but still have a bite.

If the mushrooms get dry at any point, add some more oil and a dash of soy sauce. Season with the salt, pepper and sugar to taste.

Cook the rice noodles according to the packet.

While the rice noodles are cooking, add the frozen peas to the mushroom frying pan with a nobble of vegan butter/vegetable oil and fry for 3-5 minutes.

Place the noodles into the bowls, with a few ladles of broth, a spoonful of the mushroom mix and a sprinkle of crispy tofu pieces.

Serve with the lime wedges, the greens of the spring onions, some more sliced chilli (optional)and any other toppings you might like.

Enjoy with a fork and a deep spoon.

Mum's Tomato Soup

A quick, easy peasy (hehe), hearty and healthy soup. My mum loves soup and this is always her go to.

Ingredients

1 onion, finely chopped

½ tablespoon oil

1 clove of garlic (optional)

1 carrot, sliced

6 large tomatoes, halved and sprinkled with a little salt and sugar

1 stock cube, dissolved in 600ml water

About 200g of red lentils, rinsed

A dash or two of apple cider vinegar

Handful of fresh basil, chopped

Season to taste

Method

Fry the onion in the oil, on a medium heat, until it is soft and light brown (roughly 10 mins).

Add the garlic and fry until soft (a few mins).

Add the carrots and fry for a minute or two.

Add the tomatoes, stir it all around to coat everything in the mixture.

Add the stock.

Add the lentils.

Add the cider vinegar, then bring to the boil, lower the heat and simmer for 30 minutes.

Add the chopped basil.

Season with salt and pepper.

Blend with a hand/stick blender.

Serve and enjoy.

It will keep in the fridge in a Tupperware microwaveable pot for a few days. Reheat in the microwave for 3 minutes.

It is also good if you put it into individual portions and freeze them for up to 2 months. Perfect for when you need a quick, warming lunch.

SIMPLE SUPPERS - *for those working days when you just want to knock up a quick dish with little washing up, reheat some leftovers, or pull something out of the freezer.*

I've made a few codes 🖑 = super quick, 🖑🖑= a little longer and 🖑🖑🖑= even longer still.

Ⓗ = can be reheated in the microwave usually 4 minutes per portion.

❀ = can be frozen up to one month.

'Tuna' Pasta 🖐 Ⓗ

Serves 3

Boil **300 of penne pasta** in heavily salted water (it should taste like sea water) for 8-10 minutes, depending on how al dente you like your pasta.

While the pasta is cooking, prepare the faux tuna -

1 tin of **chickpeas/haricot beans**, drained

75g of **vegan mayo**

1 heaped tbsp of **capers** + 1 tsp of **caper brine**

1 tbsp of **nutritional yeast**

½ sheet of **nori**, crumpled into small pieces (optional, but helps give a fishy taste)

1½ tsp of **salt**

Pinch of **black pepper**

Dash of **vegan Worcester sauce**

½ tsp of **white vinegar**

Juice of **1 lemon**

Optional: **1 tsp of miso paste**.

Mash ingredients together with a fork or a potato masher and mix in 1 tin **(200g) of sweetcorn**.

I also like to add **50g peas per person.**

Drain the pasta, mix with the 'tuna' and enjoy

Alternatively -

Marigold makes a vegan 'tunah' that you can buy in the co-op if you live in Wales.

You can also buy it on Amazon, so that could be used on days where you want minimal effort, just add any of the above ingredients to suit your taste. You get about 3 sandwiches worth of tuna in each tin, so it comes out at about £1 per serving, which is expensive, but I promise you, it is JUST like tuna.

Loaded Pesto Pasta 🖐️🖐️ Ⓗ

Serves 6

Many shop bought pestos contain parmesan which is made using one of the stomachs of a calf to curdle the milk. This means that most shop bought pesto isn't even vegetarian, so why not make an even more delicious version at home, which is parmesan free? You can also add some fresh baby spinach/rocket or other greens when making the pesto to make it even more nutritious.

Ingredients

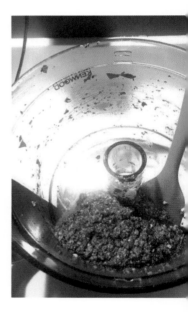

400-600g of fusilli pasta (depending on how hungry you are)

1 garlic clove

100g basil

50g cashews (feel free to omit these if you're nut free, could substitute for some sunflower seeds)

50g pine nuts (you can also omit these if you're allergic)

Splash of extra v olive oil

Dash of lemon juice

A sprinkle of sugar and lots of s & p

Method

Deskin and crush the garlic clove with the heel of your palm on the flat of a knife and leave to sit

Cook the pasta according to the pack.

While the pasta is cooking, blitz together the other ingredients (including the garlic) in a food processor. Add water to reach your desired consistency.

I like to add a cup of frozen peas or some green beans or some broccoli florets to the boiling pasta water in the last 3 minutes of cooking to make the meal a bit more filling.

Drain the pasta (and peas if you added any) and mix in the pesto.
At this point, I like to add about **20 black olives**, crushed in half, **6 large sundried tomatoes**, cut into slices, and **200g of hulled hemp hearts** (for protein). But feel free to keep it simple.

If you don't like the texture of the hemp hearts, add them into the pesto so that they get blended up.

This pesto freezes really well so we like to make it in batches and always have some in the freezer.

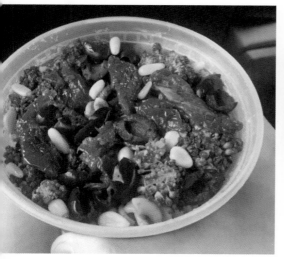 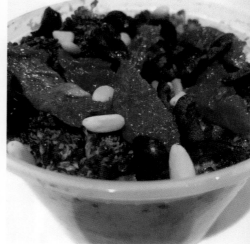

Cashew and Spinach Pasta 🖐🖐 Ⓗ

Serves 6

When I'm at uni I like to boil some water while I'm having my breakfast and pour it into a bowl of cashew nuts before I leave the house. This allows the cashews to soak all day, making them really soft when I get home, ready for me to blend to make a fast and delicious meal.

Ingredients

400g of cashew nuts (or shelled sunflower seeds if you're nut free)

1 vegetable stock cube

380ml of water (for making the sauce, not for soaking)

400-600g of farfalle (any pasta will do I just like the bows)

12 blocks of frozen spinach

Lots of salt and pepper

Method

Pour some boiling water into a bowl with the cashew nuts and the stock cube and leave for at least 2 hours (the longer the better if your blender isn't that strong).

If you're in a rush, you can boil the cashews on the hob for 30 mins.

Cook the pasta according to the instructions on the pack.

While the pasta is cooking, scoop the cashew nuts out of the water and into a blender, with a little of the 380ml of water and blend.

If you want it really smooth, make sure you're using a blender (i.e. the thing for smoothies), or a stick blender rather than a food processor (the thing for hummus), but it really doesn't have to be too smooth.

Keep adding the water, little by little, until you achieve a smooth cream.

In the last 3 minutes of the pasta's cook time, add the frozen spinach into the boiling water to defrost.

Once the pasta is cooked to your liking, drain and mix in the cashew cream.

Season to taste (I like to make it quite peppery but that's personal preference) and enjoy.

Warning, I really like spinach, so you might find that you need less spinach for your family but play around and adjust it until it's right for you.

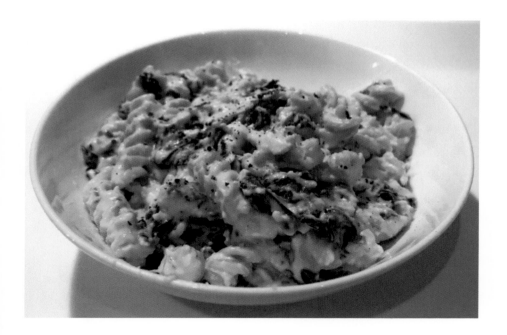

Spaghetti Bolognese 🖐🖐 Ⓗ ❄

Serves 6

This spag bol is not very traditional but it is very delicious and a real favourite in my house. It may take a little time the first few times you make it but when you get used to the recipe you can do it pretty quickly.

Ingredients

3 aubergines, diced

1 onion, diced

5 cloves of garlic, minced

2 sprigs of fresh rosemary, finely chopped, or 1 tsp dried

2 tsp paprika

2 tsp of fennel seeds, ground

Handful of fresh parsley, roughly chopped, or 2 tsp dried

Handful of fresh basil, roughly chopped, or 2 tsp dried. *Alternatively, you can use 2 tsp of homemade pesto (pg 56)*

2 red peppers, chopped into bite size chunks

30 black olives, crushed in half using your hands

½ tube of tomato puree (you don't have to use this much; I just like it really tomatoey)

300ml of tomato passata/a tin of tomatoes

1.5 mugs (350g) of uncooked, rinsed brown/puy lentils. *Or, if you're in a rush, you can use pre-cooked lentils, or frozen vegan mince.*

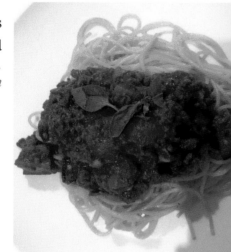

A few dashes of vegan Worcester sauce

Dash of soy sauce

Juice of 1 lemon

1-2 tsp of sugar

Salt and pepper

600g of dried spaghetti

Extra virgin olive oil for drizzling

Method

Fry the aubergine pieces with the onions in 3 tbsp of sunflower/olive oil on a medium heat for about 10 minutes, until the onions are going translucent and the aubergine is browning.

Add the garlic, rosemary, paprika, fennel and basil and heat until fragrant (if you're using dried basil and parsley add now too).

If the pan is getting dry, add a splash of oil or water to stop anything sticking.

Add in the red peppers, olives, tomato puree, passata, lentils and 500ml of water and bring to the boil. After it has come to the boil, reduce to a simmer and cook the lentils for 30-50 minutes, depending on the cooking instructions on the pack, with the lid on.

Don't forget to regularly check to ensure there is enough water in the pan to cook the lentils.

Top tip: salt can make lentils quite firm, regardless of how long you cook them for, so always try to add salt at the end when cooking with lentils.

(If you are using precooked lentils/vegan mince, only add 200 ml of water and simmer for 15 minutes. If you like your peppers soft, cook the sauce for 15 minutes before adding the mince/cooked lentils).

While the sauce is cooking, cook the spaghetti for 8 minutes in heavily salted water and drizzle with extra virgin olive oil after draining.

When the lentils are soft, but still hold their shape, (add in the fresh herbs/pesto if using) and use the soy sauce, Worcester sauce, jest and juice of a lemon, sugar and salt and pepper to adjust the flavours to your taste.

Serve with the spaghetti, the minted peas (pg 149) and a sprinkle of vegan cheese or nutritional yeast.

Lasagne using Leftover Bolognese Sauce

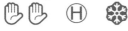

Serves 6

Lasagne may seem intimidating or far too much work for a weeknight meal, however, we like to make it in the same week that we make the spag bol so the leftovers can be used. This means that all you have to do is make a quick and easy bechamel and assemble.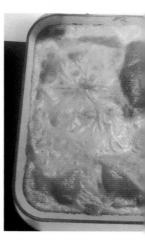

Ingredients

Leftover spag bol (different amounts needed for different sized dishes, we use a 30 x 28 x 8cm dish, which can be filled by about 4 portions of leftovers)

3 tbsp of vegan butter or olive oil

2 tbsp of plain flour

500ml of unsweetened soya milk (you can use other milks; however, it will affect the taste of the bechamel so try to choose a fairly neutral milk)

If you're scaling this, the plain flour must always be 1 tbsp less than the oil, i.e. 6 tbsp oil, 5 tbsp flour, 1000 ml milk

Generous pinch of nutmeg

2 tbsp of nutritional yeast

Squeeze of lemon

Plenty of salt and pepper

Lasagne sheets

Vegan cheese

Method

Preheat the oven to 200°C/180°C fan and put the dish that you're using into the oven to preheat.

Melt the vegan butter/heat the oil to a medium high heat in a saucepan.

Add the flour and stir thoroughly to ensure that it's all mixed in. Cook for 3 minutes.

Turn up the heat and add the milk little by little, whisking constantly to stop any lumps forming.

Once the bechamel has simmered for a few minutes it should be a good thickness to pour onto your lasagne.

Take off the heat and grate in some fresh nutmeg, squeeze in the lemon juice and generously season to taste.

It is worth pouring a small glass of the milk you're using and adding some lemon juice in advance to check that it doesn't curdle or split

Take the dish out of the oven, with gloves on and prepare for assembly. The order I like to do is: oil, lasagne sheets, Bolognese sauce, sheets, bol sauce, sheets, and then finish with a thick layer of bechamel, grated cheese/stringy cheese sauce (pg 120) and salt and pepper.

If your spag bol is a not overly saucy, add a tin of tomatoes/extra water as the pasta will absorb liquid.

Put the dish into the oven for 40 minutes, until the lasagne sheets are soft and serve with any of the delicious salads in this book (pg 40) and some oven chips.

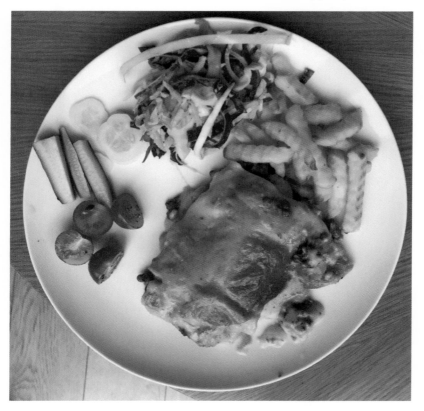

Spinach and Sausage Penne 🖐 Ⓗ

Serves 6

Ingredients

400-600g of penne pasta

600g of your favourite vegan sausages, chopped into small pieces

3 garlic cloves, crushed

2 tsp paprika

½ tsp of cayenne pepper (can add more if you fancy it spicy)

330g of cherry tomatoes, halved

1 tin of tomatoes

10 blocks of frozen spinach or 5 large handfuls of fresh spinach

Salt and pepper

Handful of black olives, crushed **OPTIONAL**

Extra virgin olive oil

Method

Start by cooking your penne pasta in a heavily salted pan of boiling water for about 8 minutes.

While the pasta is cooking, fry your sausage pieces in a frying pan with a little oil on a medium heat, for about 7 minutes or until they're going golden.

If your sausages are frozen, cook them whole in the frying pan until they are soft enough to cut into pieces and then do the step above.

Add the garlic and the spices to the pan and fry for a few minutes until they are fragrant.

Add the halved cherry tomatoes and turn the heat up a little, allowing them to blister, but not go mushy.

If the pan is getting dry, add a dash of water.

Mix in the tinned tomatoes and spinach and cook until the spinach has defrosted.

Season with salt and pepper to taste.

If you use inexpensive tinned tomatoes, they can sometimes taste a little bitter so this can be combated with a squeeze of lime juice and a sprinkle of sugar.

Drain the pasta and return it to the saucepan with a drizzle of olive oil.

Mix in the sausage and tomato sauce, sprinkle in the olives (if doing) and serve.

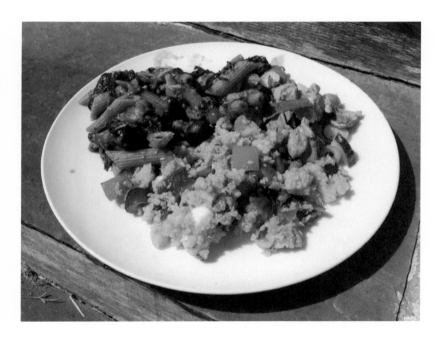

Spaghetti Carbonara 🖐🖐 Ⓗ

Serves 6

Ingredients

2 tbsp vegan butter (feel free to use oil, I just think butter adds a nice flavour here)

1 onion, finely diced

150g 'bacon' (you can use Quorn bacon, which is vegetarian or Quorn ham, Vivera bacon pieces or 'This isn't bacon rashers' which are vegan). If you don't want to include vegan bacon, you can slice tempeh (pg 151) into bacon rasher shape and rub with smoked paprika, salt and a little sugar, or just add some smoked paprika to the mushrooms

6 cloves of garlic, finely diced

½ tsp smoked paprika

300g mushrooms, sliced

1 mug frozen peas

For the Sauce

100g cashew nuts (soaked if you have a weaker blender). You can sub this for sunflower seeds if you're nut free, if you avoid seeds too, add a little flour instead to help thicken the sauce

1 block silken tofu (349g). This is just to add protein and make the dinner more filling, if you don't have any tofu/don't want to include it, that's fine but you might have to adjust the amount of liquid added

270ml non-dairy milk (unsweetened soya has the mildest flavour but if you're avoiding soya milk for any reason, feel free to use others)

4 tbsp nutritional yeast

1-2 tsp sugar

Dash soy sauce (use gf if necessary)

Dash vegan Worcester sauce

Dash of apple cider vinegar

Salt & pepper

¼ - ½ tsp of black salt/kala namak **OPTIONAL**, to give an eggy taste - use sparingly

To Serve

450g dried spaghetti (feel free to use gf if you need to)

Handful of fresh parsley

Method

Heat the vegan butter in the pan and fry the onions on a medium heat for 10 minutes.

Meanwhile, cook the 'bacon' according to the instructions on the packet (although, I personally find that grilling veggie bacon/ham results in a much better texture). This is a good time to cook the pasta.

Once the onions are soft and beginning to caramelise, add the garlic, mushrooms and smoked paprika and cook for a further 5 minutes.

While the mushrooms are cooking, blend together all the sauce ingredients until smooth and season to taste (be generous with the salt and pepper).

If the mushrooms are soft (but still have a bite), pour in the sauce with the peas and heat for about 5 minutes until the peas are cooked through and the sauce is hot.

Enjoy with the cooked spaghetti and a sprinkle of fresh parsley.

Carbonara pictured here with some pan fried asparagus and 'my take on bruschetta', (pg 147).

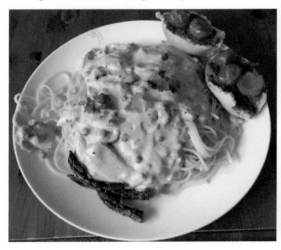

Aitken Mac 'no' Cheese ✋✋ Ⓗ

Serves 6

I adore cheese, I'd say that is the thing I've missed most since going vegan, but weirdly enough, I never used to be mad about mac 'n' cheese. I think it was just because the ones you could buy in packs used to taste like fake cheese which put me off. However, when I started dating my boyfriend, I would go to his house and his mum would make the most delicious mac 'n' cheese I'd ever had; so I have tried to replicate it here, but without any dairy. I am not going to tell you that this is some 'super authentic' mac 'n' cheese, because it's not, but I do think that it is really delicious.

Ingredients

600g dry macaroni (Tesco sell a gluten free version if necessary)

1 pack of vegan bacon of choice (you can go wild and use 2 packs if you want)

2 leeks, washed and finely sliced

3 courgettes, washed and sliced about 1cm thick

For the Sauce

4 tbsp of vegan butter or olive oil

3 tbsp of plain flour (gf works too)

3 tsp garlic powder

700-1000ml of unsweetened soya milk (you can use other milks, however, it will affect the taste of the sauce so try to choose a fairly neutral milk)

The cream from 1 tin of coconut milk/ 250ml vegan cream **OPTIONAL**, refrigerate the night before to help the cream separate.

Generous pinch of nutmeg

5 tbsp of nutritional yeast

2 level tsp Dijon mustard **OPTIONAL**

1 tsp sugar

2 tsp miso paste **OPTIONAL**

Squeeze of lemon

I would advise pouring a little milk into a glass and adding a squeeze of lemon juice in advance to check that it doesn't separate the milk.

Dash soy sauce

Dash vegan Worcester sauce

Plenty of salt and pepper

[If you want a more protein, you can blend the sauce with silken tofu, or soaked cashews, or even white beans such as broad beans]

For the Top

Vegan cheese of choice, grated, or my 'stringy cheese sauce' from pg 120 (I like to use a combination of vegan cheddar and vegan mozzarella.

Breadcrumbs/ hemp seeds to give a crunchy top **OPTIONAL**

Fresh basil and thyme, finely chopped **OPTIONAL**

Thin slices of tomatoes **OPTIONAL**

Method

Cook the vegan bacon according to the instructions on the packet. I would recommend grilling as that will produce the driest bacon, if you fry it can often go soggy in the mac 'n' cheese.

Meanwhile, fry the courgettes and leeks in a frying pan over a medium heat, with 2 tbsp oil for 15 minutes, or until lightly caramelised.

While the veg is cooking, add the vegan butter, plain flour and garlic powder into a saucepan, and heat over a medium heat, stirring until it forms a paste.

Add the soya milk, little by little, stirring constantly, until you get your desired consistency. If you want to thicken it more, bring to a simmer and simmer for 5-10 minutes. It helps to use a whisk here to ensure that there are no lumps. Don't worry if it is a little runny, it will thicken up in the oven as the pasta absorbs the sauce.

Add all the other sauce ingredients to the saucepan and stir to combine. Taste the sauce, if you want it cheesier, add more nutritional yeast and miso paste, if you want it more savoury, add more Worcester sauce etc. You must taste and adjust now because if you leave it until the end, it will be very difficult to add the seasoning and you'll end up with a bland mac 'n' cheese.

Preheat the oven to 220°C/200°C fan.

Cook the macaroni in salted boiling water, in a very large saucepan, for around 6 minutes, you don't want them to be fully cooked or you will get a mushy mac 'n' cheese.

Drain the pasta and put it back into the saucepan.

Pour the sauce into the saucepan and add the vegetables and the bacon. Give it a thorough stir to ensure that it is all coated, then pour into an ovenproof dish. Sprinkle any toppings you'd like over the top.

Bake in the oven for 20-30 minutes, or until golden brown and crispy on top. Alternatively, you can grill on a low heat for 5-10 minutes, if you do this, I recommend cooking the macaroni for a little longer as it has less time to cook under the grill.

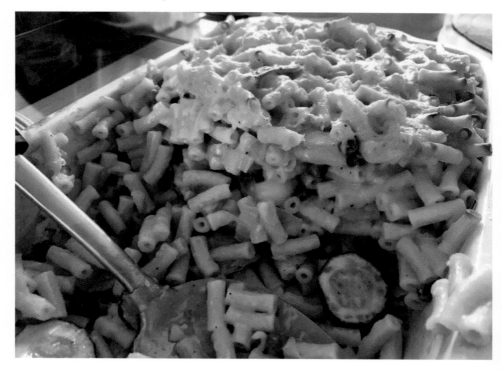

Jacket Potato Fillings ✋

To cook the potato

Don't forget to perforate the potatoes generously to allow steam to escape

	Ordinary Potato (1 serving)	Sweet Potato (1 serving)
Microwave	Cook for 8-10 minutes on full heat, flipping and drying with a paper towel halfway through the cooking time.	Cook for 5-7 minutes on full heat, flipping and drying halfway.
Oven 220°C/200°C fan	Rub the outside with a high temperature cooking oil (like vegetable) and a little salt and cook at for 1 hour - 1 hour 20 mins, depending on the size of the potato.	Cook for 40 minutes - 1 hour, depending on the size of the potato.

Check that the potatoes are fully cooked by stabbing with a sharp knife, it should be able to go through with ease.

Microwaving the potatoes is obviously a lot faster, however, you won't get the same crispy skin so you can bake in the oven for 15-20 mins at 200°C, or grill on high for a few minutes if you want the best of both worlds.

If you are microwaving multiple potatoes at once, a good rule of thumb is to multiply the time taken by 1.6 for every extra potato.

E.g. microwaving 3 jacket potatoes at once will take 8 x 1.6 x 1.6 = 20.5 minutes.

Top tip - If you are cooking in the oven and want little clean up, line the baking tray with tin foil in advance as the potatoes tend to weep a bit (kind of sinister, I know).

Pulled BBQ Jackfruit *Serves 6*	Hummus and Veg *Serves 6*	Refried Beans *Serves 6*
Ingredients 1 onion, finely diced 5 cloves of garlic, minced 1 tsp paprika 2 tsp smoked paprika 1 tsp cayenne pepper (optional) 2½ tbsp brown sugar/maple syrup 8 tbsp tomato puree 2 tins of jackfruit, drained ½ tsp apple cider vinegar 1 tbsp soy sauce 1 tbsp vegan Worcester sauce 2 tsp Dijon mustard **(OPTIONAL)** Salt and pepper	**Ingredients** 3 red peppers 2 carrots, peeled into thin slithers 600g hummus (bought or homemade, (pg 157) Sprinkle of sesame seeds, if you want Garnish with any greenery you have, i.e. spring onions, watercress	**Ingredients** 1 onion, diced 3 cloves of garlic, minced 2 green peppers, cut into small pieces 2 chillies (optional), cut into slices 2 tins of pinto beans, drained Squeeze of lime Handful of fresh coriander, roughly chopped Silken tofu sour cream (pg 123)
Method Fry the onion, garlic, spices and sugar in ½ tbsp of sunflower oil, on a medium-low heat for 10-15 minutes, allowing the onions to caramelise. While the onions are cooking, shred the jackfruit into pulled pork-esque strips.	**Method** If you're having this in winter, it is delicious with the red peppers roasted, however, in summer it is lovely and refreshing with raw red peppers. (If roasting) Cook the peppers, with a generous drizzle of oil and a sprinkle of salt and pepper, in the oven	**Method** Fry the onion, garlic, green peppers, and chillies with 1 tbsp of oil on a medium-low heat for 10 minutes until the onions are starting to caramelise. Add both tins of pinto beans, turn up the heat and fry for a minute or two then add a little

Add the tomato puree, jackfruit, vinegar, Worcester sauce, mustard and soy sauce to the onions, with enough water to cover the jackfruit.

Ideally simmer for around 40 minutes (20 mins minimum) until the jackfruit melts in the mouth and you have a sticky and delicious sauce.

If it gets too dry at any point, add a dash of water.

Season with salt and pepper to taste.

If you can't find jackfruit, you can shred oyster mushrooms for a similar result. If you want to save time, cook the jackfruit in a bought BBQ sauce.

for 20 minutes at 220°C/200°C fan.

After the peppers are done, assemble on top of a hot jacket potato and enjoy.

water and simmer for 10 minutes.

After they are heated through, mush the beans a little with a fork.

Serve with plenty of blobs of sour cream and a sprinkle of fresh coriander.

Other fillings

- Faux tuna from the 'tuna pasta' recipe on pg 55
- Baked beans with vegan cheese (a classic)
- Tapenade (pg 159) with blistered cherry tomatoes (pg 147) and caramelised red onion (pg 149)
- Chilli sin carne (pg 114)
- To bring out the flavour of the sweet potato I like to slather some butter on the inside and mix in a sprinkle of cinnamon and the zest of a lime

Mushroom Tagliatelle ✋ Ⓗ

This is a simple, super quick, one pan dish to make. Serve with your favourite pasta and some lovely green vegetables.

Ingredients

2 tbsp sunflower oil

2 onions, finely diced

500g mushrooms, sliced

3 cloves of garlic, crushed

400ml unsweetened oat milk

Silken tofu (optional extra if extra protein is required)

2 large tbsp plain flour - (I use gluten free)

Nutmeg

Fresh thyme, rosemary, and oregano

Salt and pepper

2 tbsp vegan cream (I like Alpro single soya)

2 tbsp nutritional yeast

Method

Add half of the chopped onion to a frying pan on a medium-high heat and sauté in the oil for about 10 minutes until soft, sweet and light brown.

Add the sliced mushrooms and other half of the chopped onions to the frying pan.

Stir, coating all the mushrooms and onions with the oil, add more oil if necessary.

Fry on a medium heat with the lid on for another 10 minutes.

Add the flour to the frying pan.

Add a handful of chopped fresh herbs - rosemary, thyme, oregano.

Stir to coat all the ingredients with the flour and cook for a couple of minutes until you can't see the flour anymore.

Add salt and pepper and ¼ teaspoon of ground nutmeg.

Slowly add up to 400ml of oat milk (you don't have to add it all), stirring frequently. As the mixture warms up it will start to thicken. Add enough oat milk until you get a slightly thicker than required consistency.

Top tip - if you are very hungry and have done lots of exercise; add less of the oat milk and blend (hand blender is ideal) a pack of silken tofu until it is smooth and add this to your mixture - it will add extra protein.

Just before you serve, pour in a couple of tablespoons of vegan cream and a couple of tablespoons of nutritional yeast.

Meanwhile cook your favourite pasta and green veg to accompany.

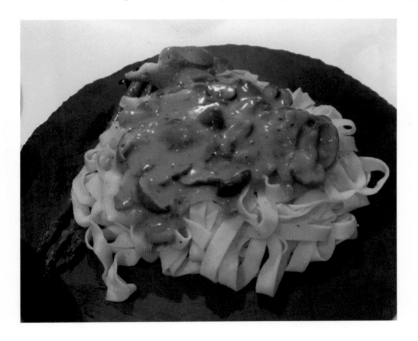

Dad's Roast Mushroom and Vegetable Pie 🖐🖐 Ⓗ

Serves 6

In our house my mum thinks her pie is best, but my dad thinks his is...what do you think?

Ingredients

2 large punnets of button mushrooms, quartered

1 butternut squash peeled, deseeded and chopped into bite size pieces

2 peppers - whatever colour you have- chopped

1 large sweet potato, chopped into bite size pieces (roughly 2cm cubes)

Any other vegetables that you fancy roasting

2 large onions, finely chopped

2 garlic cloves, crushed

1 tbsp brown sugar

A good amount of thyme and rosemary - fresh if you have it but dried if not

Heaped tbsp of flour, gluten free if required

300ml vegetable stock

2 tbsp soy sauce

Heaped tbsp grainy mustard (optional but my Dad likes it)

Pastry topping - either readymade or homemade

Method

Preheat the oven to 200°C/ 180°C fan.

Chop the mushrooms, squash, peppers, potato, and anything else that you fancy roasting, into bite sized pieces.

Put these in 2 baking trays, add a generous glug of sunflower/vegetable oil, mix and roast for 30 minutes, turning once.

Meanwhile, fry the onions until starting to caramelise (about 10 minutes on a medium heat).

Add the garlic, sugar, thyme and rosemary and cook really gently until it looks golden and delicious - maybe about 10 minutes.

Add the flour and stir well to ensure that everything is coated.

Slowly add the stock and stir to ensure that no lumps form - you should have a nice thick and smooth gravy.

Add the soy sauce and roasted vegetables and stir gently to give a lovely thick, aromatic and colourful pie filling.

Pour the mixture into an ovenproof dish and top with your pastry. I like to make a design on the top to show it some love. Cook in the oven for around 30 minutes.

Boom - the BEST pie ever! (My Dad wrote this recipe haha).

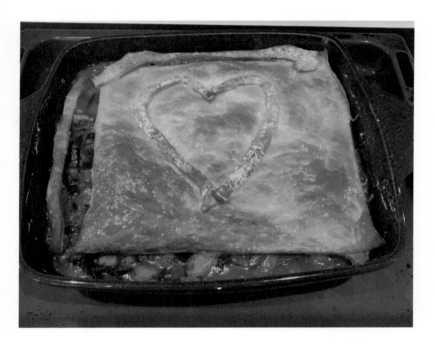

Shepherd's Pie 🖐🖐🖐

Serves 6

A family dish going back generations - however NEVER before was it plant based… but here we go; and we think it's just as yummy.

Ingredients

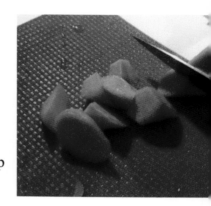

<u>For the Mash</u>

2.5kg of Maris Piper potatoes, quartered

3 tbsp vegan butter

A dash of unsweetened oat/hemp milk

Some grated vegan mature cheddar for the top

<u>For the Sauce</u>

1 onion, finely diced

1 celery, finely chopped (roughly 1mm)

6 carrots, cut into diagonal chunks (see page opposite)

250g button mushrooms, quartered

500g bag of frozen meat free mince (alternatively you can use lentils, see pg 24)

2 tablespoons of plain flour (I use gluten free)

A large handful of fresh rosemary, thyme and sage, chopped

½ tsp nutritional yeast

Soy sauce (can use gluten free)

Worcester sauce

4 tbsp tomato ketchup

2 stock cubes

Accompaniments

Beetroot

Pickled red cabbage

Frozen peas

Method:

Peel the potatoes (don't have to if you are feeling lazy), chop into quarters (3cm squares), add to a large saucepan and then cover with water (don't cook yet).

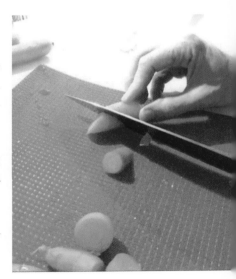

Finely chop the onion and add to a frying pan with a tablespoon of oil. Fry on a low/medium heat.

Wash the celery, top and tail; then thinly slice and add to the onions.

Fry for about 10 minutes on a medium heat until the onions are soft and light brown.

Add some salt and pepper.

Wash and chop the carrots, then add to the frying pan.

Cook for 10 minutes with the lid on.

Wash and chop the mushrooms, add to the pan with the herbs, stir well, replace the lid and cook for another 10 minutes.

Meanwhile drain the potatoes and replace with some fresh water (this removes excess starch), bring the potatoes to the boil, add a pinch of salt and boil for 20 minutes or until the potatoes are soft.

Now, add the flour to the frying pan, stir until you can't see it anymore. Add a crumbled stock cube, slowly add about 350ml of water or until the mixture is a nice lightly thick consistency. Add a couple of dashes of Worcester sauce, soy sauce and the tomato ketchup.

When you have a nice, rich, saucy sauce, add the vegan mince. Stir well.

Put the empty casserole dish in the oven 200°C/180°C fan to warm it up.

By this time, the potatoes should be cooked. Drain the water off, add the butter and oat milk to the still warm saucepan and mash until smooth and creamy.

Take the pan out of the oven (don't burn yourself!), pour the vegetable sauce into the dish, spoon the mash potato into blobs all over the top of the sauce and then lightly use a fork to spread the mash out.

Grate some cheese on the top and put it into the oven for 30 - 40 minutes. For extra deliciousness, place it under the grill for a few minutes to brown the cheese just before serving.

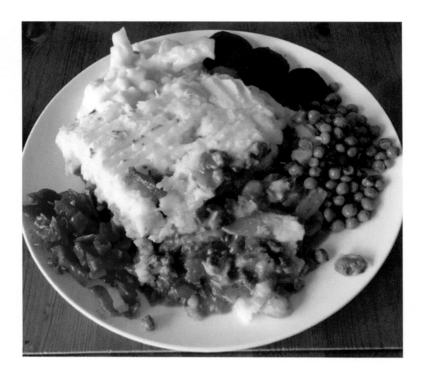

Leek and Mushroom Pie 🖐🖐 Ⓗ

Serves 6

Which do you prefer, this or the roast vegetable pie on pg 76?

Top tip: double the recipe and have it for leftovers the next day.

Ingredients

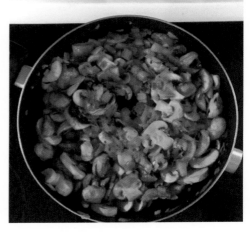

4 leeks, sliced to about 2cm thick

1 onion, finely sliced

500g assorted mushrooms, sliced

4 cloves garlic, finely chopped

2-3tbsp plain flour (can use gf)

500ml oat milk

1 stock cube

2 tbsp soya single cream

Readymade gluten free puff pastry (we have tried, many times, to make our own vegan and gluten free pastry, but none of them have ever compared to the "Jus-Rol" one that you can get in the supermarkets, if you want to make your own, go for it, but if you just want a quick dinner, we'd advise buying it)

A sprinkle of nutritional yeast

Salt, pepper, nutmeg, fresh rosemary fresh thyme

Sunflower oil

Method

Wash 4 leeks thoroughly and slice (leeks can often have sand in their inner layers so make sure you wash all the inside too).

Add to the frying pan, along with the finely sliced onion.

Add 1 tablespoon of sunflower oil.

Then turn on the heat and gently fry until soft - stirring occasionally.

Add a few twists or shakes of salt and black pepper, and ¼ teaspoon of grated nutmeg. Top tip: too much ground nutmeg is poisonous.

Meanwhile, wash and slice the mushrooms.

Then add ½ tbsp more cooking oil to the frying pan if it's a little dry, my mum likes to use Carotino's Healthier Cooking Oil.

Add the garlic to the frying pan and let it cook for a few more minutes until the garlic is soft.

Then add the chopped mushrooms.

Stir into the mixture.

Turn the heat down.

Put the lid on the frying pan.

Cook for another 10 minutes or until the mushrooms are soft.

Remove the lid, stir and check the mushrooms are soft.

Preheat the oven to 240°C /220°C fan.

Then add 2 tablespoons of plain flour and stir until you can't see the flour anymore.

Add some fresh thyme and rosemary to the sauce.

Add oat milk a little at a time, stirring until it's all mixed in and thickening up, you may have to turn the heat up a notch. It will require about 500ml of oat milk.

Top tip: If you want a bit more protein, whisk a packet of silken tofu in with the milk before you add it to the pan.

Crumble in the stock cube and add 2 tablespoons of single soy cream.

Get the (Gluten free) puff pastry out of the fridge to warm up a little.

If the sauce is too runny, let it simmer on the stove without a lid. This'll reduce the mixture by evaporating any water.

Sprinkle Nutritional Yeast (Engevita) over the sauce and stir in.

Pour the mixture into a 30 x 28 x 8 pie dish, roll the pastry on top and place in the oven.

Serve with some minted peas (pg 149) and oven chips and you've got yourself a fabulous dinner.

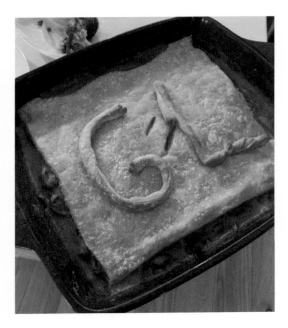

We put "GL" on this pie to stand for good luck as we made it the day before my brother's and my exams were starting.

Thai Curry 🖐️🖐️ Ⓗ

Serves 6

Ingredients

1 block of firm tofu, squeezed (pg 22) and chopped into bite size pieces (**OPTIONAL** but a good source of protein)

150g of cashew nuts (**OPTIONAL**)

1 large onion, cut into moons (like a chocolate orange)

4 cloves of garlic, finely chopped

6cm of ginger, finely chopped

2 chillies, chopped (optional)

Alternatively, if you're cooking for a family, just take the top off the chillies and cook them whole in the sauce, they can then be served to anyone who wants some extra spice, while keeping the rest of the dinner mild for anyone who isn't a fan of heat

8 carrots, cut into batons

1 tbsp lemongrass paste (a good fish sauce substitute)

1 tbsp soy sauce

½ tbsp of brown sugar

2 tins of coconut milk

Juice of 2 limes

I like to zest the limes as well so that if the sauce isn't 'limey' enough when I taste it at the end, I can just chuck in the zest

2 tins of banana blossom, drained (has an amazingly fishy texture and can be found in Sainsburys and Asda) **OPTIONAL**

1 nori sheet **OPTIONAL** (if you're going for a Thai 'fish' curry, nori really helps to give that fishy taste)

300g of mushrooms (I like the frozen mushroom medley from Tesco)

2 peppers (I like red but it's up to you), sliced (pg 16)

1 mug of frozen sweetcorn (roughly 150g)

1 mug of frozen peas/soybeans (which are just shelled edamame beans)

Salt and pepper to taste

Serve

480g uncooked basmati rice

Flaked almonds **OPTIONAL**

Bunch of fresh coriander, roughly chopped **OPTIONAL**

Method

Fry the tofu and cashew nuts in a deep frying pan with 2 tbsp of oil on a medium heat for 15 minutes, with plenty of salt and pepper. Remove the cashews if they start to get too brown

Toss regularly to ensure the tofu gets crispy on all sides. If you like your tofu really crispy, remove it from the heat now and add it as a topping at the end. If you want it to soak up the flavours, keep it in.

Add in the onion, garlic, chillies and ginger and fry with another ½ tbsp of oil on a low heat for 10 minutes. Add more oil if the pan starts to get dry.

Add all of the remaining ingredients (except peas, sweetcorn and coriander) and simmer for 20 minutes. I like my sauce to be quite thin when I'm making this dish as the rice soaks it up, but if you prefer a thicker sauce simmer with the lid off.

This is a good time to cook your rice.

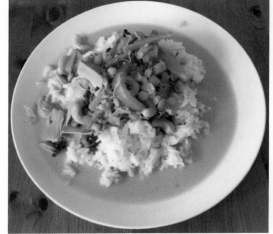

Add the frozen peas and sweetcorn and simmer for another few minutes until they are defrosted.

Taste your sauce and add lime zest, salt, pepper or sugar to taste.

Serve with cooked basmati rice, brown rice or quinoa and a sprinkle of fresh coriander and almonds.

Fried Rice 🖐

Serves 6

When I first moved into my uni house for 2nd year, the bedroom was disgusting! Dust everywhere, hair everywhere, no room to even put my suitcase down.

So, I spent the entire evening cleaning my room until it was vaguely habitable. I finished at 1am, realising that I hadn't eaten dinner, I checked out the cupboards and fridge and all that was in the house was a friend's leftover rice, some soy sauce and a singular egg!

My dinner that evening was very questionable? Luckily, since then, I have improved my fried rice recipe and made it vegan, I hope you like it.

Ingredients

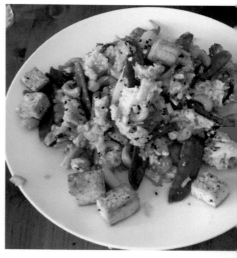

1 block of firm tofu, *squeezed* (pg 22) and cut into 2x2x2cm cubes

75g cashew nuts **OPTIONAL** (if you're nut free, sunflower seeds can add the same nice crunch)

2 tsp turmeric

2 tsp curry powder

2 tsp black onion seeds

3 cloves of garlic, finely chopped

2 courgettes, thinly sliced like 50p coins

1 broccoli, cut into bite size florets

225g of green beans, fresh or frozen, with then ends removed and chopped in half

Roughly 700g cooked and cooled basmati rice (this is the perfect dish to use up leftover rice). Top tip - You want the rice to cool as quickly as possible so it's good to spread it out over a tray to increase the surface area and then use it within 1 day of being stored in the fridge.

100g mangetout, cut in half diagonally

2 tbsp nutritional yeast

½ tsp black salt **OPTIONAL**

3 tbsp of soy sauce (or more, be generous)

2 chillies chopped **OPTIONAL**

Salt and pepper to taste

Method

Fry the tofu and cashews in 2 tbsp of sunflower oil with plenty of salt and pepper on a medium heat for 10 minutes.

Add the turmeric, curry powder, black onion seeds and garlic, turn the heat up and cook for a few minutes. Add in the broccoli, courgettes and beans with a splash of water and cook on high for about 5 minutes with the lid on.

Add in the rice and toss to ensure it is well mixed with the veg and spice. Make sure you add a bit of oil if needed and stir fry for 5 minutes, or until the rice is piping hot and lightly fried.

Finally stir in the other ingredients and serve.

Top tip: this works best with rice that has very little starch so ensure that you have rinsed VERY thoroughly and only stirred once when cooking.

Also, don't worry if the veg is still crunchy when eating, this dish is supposed to highlight the freshness of the veg, feel free to cook the veg for longer though if you'd prefer them softer.

If you don't have any precooked rice, fry the spices, garlic, courgettes, broccoli and tofu first, then add in the (thoroughly rinsed) rice to toast it, then add enough water to cover the rice and simmer with the lid on for around 15 minutes, on a low heat, and you will get a dish that's a bit more like a jambalaya, but it'll still be delicious.

Su's Stir Fry 🖐🖐 Ⓗ

Serves 6

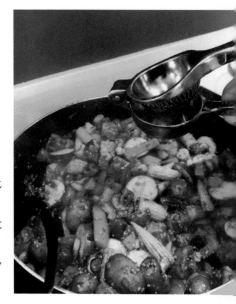

Ingredients

Salt and pepper

Neutral sunflower cooking oil (~ 5 tbsp)

6-10 drops Sesame Oil

396g pack firm tofu, squeezed (pg 22) & cut into cubes

1 white onion, peeled & cut into crescent moon shapes (pg 14)

A nobble (~6 cm) of ginger, finely chopped

4 cloves of garlic, finely chopped

150g cashew nuts

A 130g packet of baby-corn, each snapped in half

2 carrots, cut into batons

1 tbsp apple cider vinegar

2 limes, zested and juiced

1 tbsp sesame seeds

500g mushrooms, halved or sliced

2 courgettes, sliced

1 chilli, topped and sliced

1 tsp honey/ sugar

½ tbsp vegan Worcester sauce

1 tbsp soy sauce (can use gf)

2 peppers, chopped into medium-small pieces (see pg 16 for de-seeding)

1 broccoli, cut into florets

2 handfuls of French beans - top, tailed and halved

2 handfuls of mangetouts

Method

Chop the tofu as shown on pg 153. Chuck into a frying pan on a medium-high heat, with the oil and a generous helping of salt and pepper, turning regularly. After 20 minutes, the tofu should be crispy. Remove and place on one side. Alternatively, you could leave it in the sauce to soak up the flavours, however, it will be less crispy at the end. Another alternative, cook the tofu in the oven (pg 153) while you cook the rest of the stir fry.

Fry the onion slices with a tablespoon of oil for 10 minutes on a medium/high heat.

Add the chopped garlic and ginger, turn the heat down to medium-low, and cook for 5 minutes. Add extra oil if it's looking a little dry.

On a high heat, clear a space in the middle of the pan, and add the cashew nuts.

Whilst the nuts are cooking, you can prepare the other vegetables. Don't stir the nuts until they have toasted on one side.

Once the cashews are ready, thoroughly stir in the baby-corn. Reduce the heat, add the lid and leave to cook. After a few minutes, whack in the carrots and turn the heat up.

The pan may be getting dry, so add in a sprinkle of apple cider vinegar to prevent any sticking.

After a few minutes, remove the lid. Zest the 2 limes into the pan and sprinkle in the sesame seeds.

Now add the mushrooms, and sliced courgettes. Stir everything together in the pan.

You may now add the chilli. Drizzle in some cooking honey. Dash some soy sauce and Worcester sauce into the mix, and squeeze in the juice of 1 lime.

Fry for another 5 minutes, then add the peppers and cover, to cook everything all the way through. Now, add the broccoli to the top of the frying pan, with a dash of water, for steaming.

Top Tip: Adding the broccoli to the frying pan when it's hot will retain its vibrant green colour.

Bring a large pan of water to the boil. Once ready, add the rice noodles and turn off the heat. Leave for 3 minutes, then drain and rinse in cold water.

Whilst the noodles cook, add the mangetout and beans to the frying pan. Drop in the sesame oil and extra cooking oil. Season with salt and pepper to taste. Sesame oil has quite a low smoke point, i.e. you want to add it after you've finished cooking, or it can burn.

Serve with the fresh juice of the lime squeezed on top.

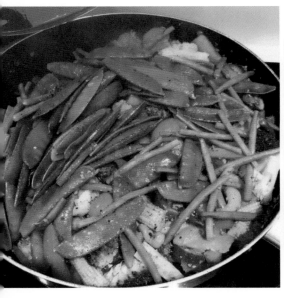
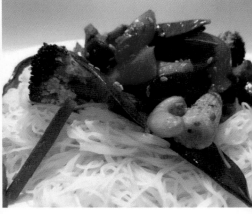

Satay Skewers 🤚🤚 Ⓗ

Serves 6

This is a really fun version of the classic chicken satay; I like to use different things on my skewers, resulting in a surprise with each bite.

In an ideal world, you would marinate the tofu in the sauce overnight, allowing the flavours to develop properly, but if you can't do that, don't worry! It still makes a quick, delicious, protein packed dinner.

Ingredients

16 BBQ skewers

1 block of firm tofu, *squeezed* (pg 22) and sliced into skewer sized cubes, roughly 3x3x3cm

The more you have squeezed the tofu, the easier it will go on the skewers

1 sweet potato, cut into the same size as the tofu

1 red onion, cut into 8ths, like a chocolate orange

2 courgettes, peeled into thin slices

6 large tomatoes, cut like a chocolate orange (into 6ths)

1 tin of coconut milk

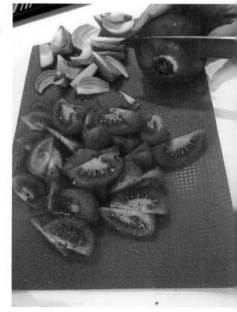

For the Satay Marinade

500g peanut butter

¾ tbsp ground turmeric

1½ tbsp ground coriander

2 tsp garlic powder

6cm fresh ginger, roughly chopped

1 hot chilli **OPTIONAL**

3 tsp lemongrass paste (1.5 sticks of lemongrass)

3 tbsp sugar

1 tin of coconut milk

2 tbsp soy sauce

Juice of 2 limes

Water

To Serve

Handful of fresh coriander (optional)

Sprinkle of flaked almonds

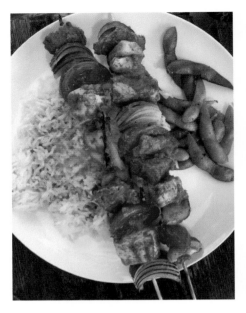

Method

Soak the skewers in warm water while you prepare the vegetables and the sauce, this will prevent them burning under the grill.

After chopping the vegetables and the tofu, put the sweet potato cubes into the microwave, in a bowl covered with cling film and microwave for about 10-15 minutes, stirring halfway.

When there are a couple of minutes left on the sweet potatoes, put the onion pieces into the bowl too, to allow them to soften.

The cooking time will vary depending on the size of the pieces, but you want the sweet potato to be cooked all the way through as they will not cook much more on the grill.

Put all the marinade ingredients into a blender and blend until smooth.

Add a little water if it's too thick and season with salt and pepper to taste.

Thread the veg and tofu onto the skewer, making a snake with the courgette slices, drizzle with oil, salt and pepper, and lay onto the grill rack, with a tray underneath to catch the sauce.

Gently pour the sauce over the skewers so that all the veg is covered and scrape the sauce that was caught by the tray into a saucepan and add the remaining tin of coconut milk.

Set the grill to high and grill the skewers for 4-7 minutes on each side. Make sure that you put the tray back under the grill rack to catch any more excess sauce while cooking.

While the skewers are cooking, you can cook some basmati rice and heat up the remaining marinade in a saucepan to deepen the flavours.

Sprinkle some flaked almonds and roughly sliced coriander on top of the skewers and serve with the basmati rice, sauce and the 'easy edamames' from pg 150.

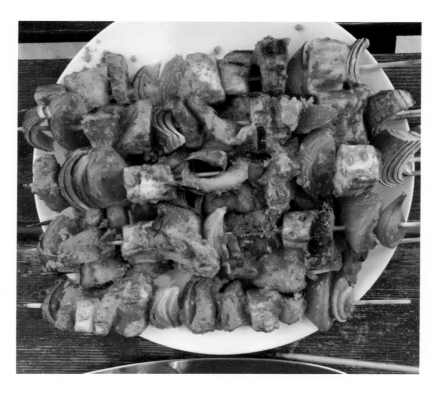

Pad Thai 🤚 Ⓗ
Serves 6

The first time I had pad Thai, I totally fell in love with it.

Peanutty, limey, just the right amount of sweetness, added to that, it's super quick to make and this version does not compromise on flavour, even without the fish sauce.

Ingredients
400g tempeh (can be found in the supermarket or see pg 151 for a recipe to make it yourself), cut into cubes

Half a white cabbage, cut into strips

2 cloves of garlic, finely chopped

4 cm ginger, finely chopped

½ block of firm tofu, squeezed (pg 22)

Either 1 tbsp nutritional yeast or ¼ tsp black salt (for an eggy flavour)

1 broccoli, cut into small florets

1 mug of frozen soybeans (shelled edamame beans)

200g mangetout

130g baby corn, cut in half lengthwise

Handful of bean sprouts

Sauce

2 tbsp lemongrass paste (a good vegan substitute for fish sauce)

2 tbsp tamarind paste (can be found in most supermarkets and all Asian supermarkets)

3 tbsp brown sugar

4 tbsp dark soy sauce (can use gf)

120g peanut butter (chunky)

1 tsp miso paste

Enough oil to make it saucy

1½ limes, juice and zest

Serving

50g peanuts

2 chillies, sliced

2-3 spring onions, sliced

1½ limes, cut into wedges

6 rice noodle nests

Method

Preheat the oven to 180°C/160°C fan.

Cut and wash all of your vegetables as the cooking hardly takes any time so you want all your veg to be ready to be thrown in.

Cut the tempeh into bite size cubes and toss in some oil, salt and pepper (can marinade overnight in soy sauce, sugar and lime if you'd like), then place on a tray in the oven for 20-25 minutes.

Place another small tray in the oven with the peanuts on and cook for 10-15 minutes or until golden brown.

Fry the cabbage in a deep frying pan with 1 tbsp of oil on a medium-high heat with a little salt, pepper and sugar for a few minutes. If the pan gets dry, add a dash of dark soy sauce.

Add the garlic and ginger and cook until the ginger is soft.

When the cabbage is softening, push it to the sides, making a hole in the middle. Crumble the squeezed, firm tofu into this hole, with the nutritional yeast/black salt, to imitate scrambled egg.

Fry for a few minutes then add in the broccoli and frozen soybeans. Add a dash of water if the pan gets too dry.

While the broccoli and beans are cooking, make your sauce by mixing together all the sauce ingredients in a jug, using vegetable oil to ensure that it is not too thick.

Boil the kettle and submerge the noodle nests in the boiled water or cook according to the instructions on the pack.

By this point, the tempeh should be nearly done, and the broccoli should be tender enough to stick a fork in, but not mushy.

Add in the mangetout, the sweetcorn, the bean sprouts and the sauce and stir to ensure everything is coated. Season with salt and pepper to taste.

Cook the sauce until everything is hot and it is the consistency that you want.

Drain the noodles and pour in with the sauce.

Serve with peanuts, chilli slices, spring onion slices and wedges of lime.

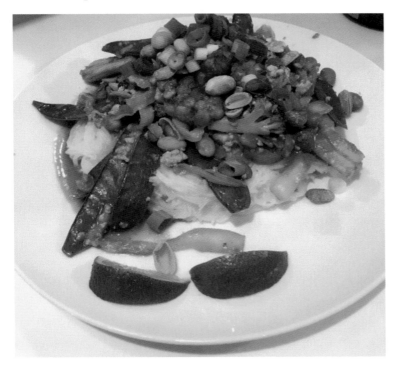

Spiced Jackfruit and Quinoa Plate ✋✋

Serves 6

This dish is always a bit of a mish-mash depending on what we have in the house at the time, but the main elements always stay the same. Don't be alarmed, I know jackfruit sounds intimidating, but it's available tinned in all the big supermarkets in the UK.

Ingredients

2 tins of young jackfruit

2 vegetable stock cubes

175g LEON chilli sauce

Can be found in Sainsburys, I like it because it is the perfect spiciness, slightly sweet and gluten free, but feel free to use a different sauce or even make your own with tomato puree, veg stock, chipotle peppers, paprika and sugar

2 cloves of garlic, finely chopped

4 large tomatoes, diced

1 carrot, diced into small cubes

1.5 mugs (300g) of quinoa, rinsed thoroughly

1 tin of black beans, drained and rinsed

Bunch of coriander, roughly chopped

2 avocados

Bunch of lettuce

(We like to serve with 'easy edamames' pg 150, roasted sweet potato pg 141, toasted cashew pg 150, roasted chickpeas pg 163, caramelised red onions pg 149 and mint yoghurt pg 122)

Method

Drain and rinse the jackfruit from the tin.

Put the jackfruit into a bowl and cover with boiling water.

Crumble in the stock cubes and stir thoroughly to ensure that the stock is dissolved.

Leave to soak for around 30 minutes.

This is a good time to prep the roasted sweet potatoes, chickpeas or any other sides you're having.

Meanwhile, heat up 1 tbsp of sunflower oil in a large saucepan and fry the garlic, tomatoes and carrots on a medium heat for 10 minutes, with the lid on, until the carrots are softening.

While the veg is frying, rinse the quinoa THOROUGHLY, either under running water for 3-5 mins (catch the water for watering plants) or in a bowl of water, regularly swirling.

Add the rinsed quinoa to the tomatoes and carrots and toast for 3-5 minutes.

Heat the oven to 200°C/180°C fan.

By now, the jackfruit should've soaked for sufficiently long, therefore you can take the jackfruit out of the bowl (making sure to keep the stock) and place it on a baking tray.

Pour 1.9 mugs worth (around 510ml) of the leftover stock into the quinoa and vegetables and bring to a simmer then reduce to low, cover and set a timer for 20 minutes.

If there isn't that much stock just add more water

Now, toss the jackfruit in 2 tbsp of sunflower oil and the LEON chilli sauce and place in the oven for 30 minutes with any other sides you may be having, don't forget to turn regularly and add more sauce if needed.

This jackfruit may stick to your baking tray, it will come off if washed, but you can always line the tray with tin foil to save time

Add the black beans to the quinoa and cook for a further 10 minutes.

Once the quinoa has finished, take it off the heat and let it sit for 5 minutes, this is a good time to start plating up.

The jackfruit which should be soft and have a similar texture to chicken.

After the quinoa has finished sitting, fluff it up with a fork, season with some salt and pepper and stir in the chopped coriander.

Serve with some fresh lettuce, sliced avocado (pg 18) and enjoy

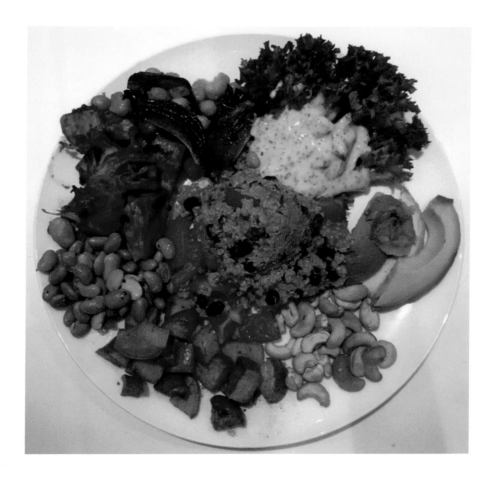

Sweet Potato Tagine 👋 Ⓗ ❄

Serves 6

This is a super simple, quick and tasty dinner. This is also a perfect dinner for using up veg that is past its best.

Ingredients

2 tbsp of cooking oil (we use sunflower or vegetable)

2 onions, cut into crescent moons (pg 14)

6 cloves garlic - whole

1 butternut squash, cut into bite size pieces

5 carrots, roughly chopped

2 red peppers, chopped (pg 16)

150g of dried apricots, halved

5 sundried tomatoes, halved

2 tins of chickpeas

1 tin of tomatoes

2 tsp paprika

1 tsp smoked paprika

1 tsp cumin

1 chilli, chopped

Dash of Worcester sauce

Dash of soy sauce

A drizzle of honey.

Extra water if you cook for a long time. + Salt n Pepper

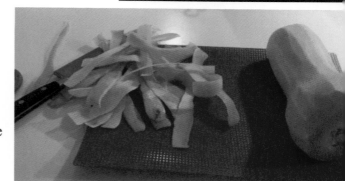

Method

Preheat the oven to 200°C/180°C fan.

Put 2 tablespoons of oil in the casserole dish.

Slice the onions like a chocolate orange, place half of them in the baking tray.

Top and tail the butternut squash, peel, cut in half lengthways, then chop into bite size pieces. When you get to the seed area, scoop out the seeds. Throw them away and carry on chopping into bite size pieces.

Place the butternut squash into the casserole dish.

Peel the garlic and add to the casserole dish.

Top and tail the carrots, then roughly chop and add to the casserole dish.

Grind some salt and pepper.

Stir well then pop in the oven for 30 minutes.

Add all the remaining ingredients (including the chickpea water).

Return to the oven for another 20 minutes.

Serve with couscous/quinoa (pg 28) with a handful of cranberries added, a sprinkling of pine nuts and spinach.

Keeps well in the fridge for 3 days, in fact the taste just gets better and better.

It can be frozen for up to a couple of months.

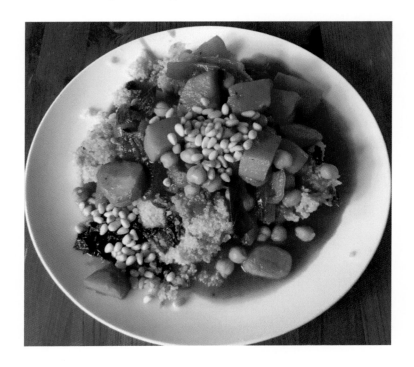

Paella 🤚🤚 Ⓗ

Serves 6

Ingredients

1 red onion, chopped into crescents (pg 14)

18 little plum tomatoes, whole

1 tbsp balsamic vinegar

6 cloves of garlic, finely chopped

2 tbsp capers, chopped/crushed into tiny pieces

1 tsp smoked paprika

2 tsp sweet paprika

1 tsp dried thyme

½ tsp cayenne pepper

1 red pepper, cut into strips

5 large white mushrooms, cut into slices

1 courgette, cut into thick slices (1cm)

100g green, pitted olives

1 sheet of nori, chopped up finely **OPTIONAL**

300g of paella rice (can be found in Sainsburys and other supermarkets, if you can't find it, feel free to use arborio or another short grain rice- long grain rice will cook, it will just take a long time)

960ml hot vegetable stock with a pinch of turmeric to give that characteristic yellow

Salt and pepper

1 mug of frozen peas

To Serve

1 lemon, cut into wedges

A handful of fresh parsley

Method

Ideally, this should be cooked in a deep frying pan that is <u>non-stick,</u> this helps to make the classic paella crust, if you don't have this it is not the end of the world, it will still taste delicious.

Fry the red onion in a frying pan, with 2 tbsp of vegetable oil, on a high heat for around 6 minutes until the moons are translucent and beginning to brown.

Add the tomatoes and cook for about 5 minutes, allowing the skin to blister, but not go mushy.

Add the balsamic vinegar to deglaze the pan.

Reduce to a medium heat and add the garlic, capers, herbs and spices and cook for around 3 minutes, until fragrant.

Add the pepper, mushrooms, courgette and olives, with a bit of oil if necessary and cook for a few minutes, ensuring they are covered in the spices.

Add about 1 tsp of salt and 1 tsp black pepper.

Turn up the heat a little and add the rice, allowing it to toast in the pan for 1-2 minutes

Then pour in the vegetable stock, but DO NOT STIR.

Stirring will bring the starch out of the rice, making it more of a creamy risotto than a paella.

Bring to a simmer and let it simmer for about 20 minutes until the rice is soft, but firm. Check that there is no liquid in the pan, if there is, simmer for a little longer.

Once cooked, remove the pan from the heat and put the frozen peas on top of the paella and cover it, allowing them to thaw. Leave the paella for 10 minutes, then serve with the parsley and lemon wedges.

If you'd like a little more protein, sprinkle my 'crispy tofu pieces' (pg 150) on top.

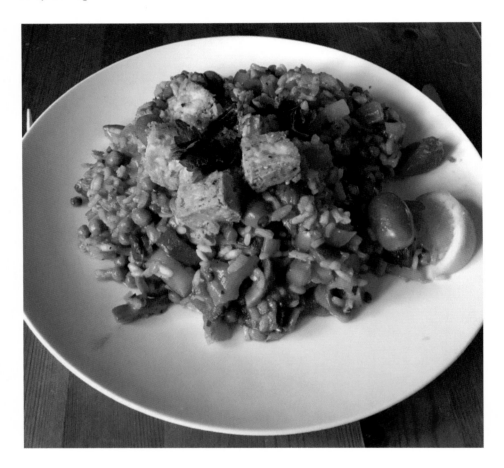

Tomato and Chorizo Jambalaya ✋ Ⓗ

Serves 6

An absolutely delicious, simple quick dish to make. Leftovers are great for the next day or two.

Not much washing up either - one large pan with a lid is all you need, oh and a spoon!

Ingredients

Tablespoon of oil	.10
280g of vegan chorizo sausages (eg Plant Pioneers Shroomdogs)	£2.50
1 onion	.10
4 sticks of celery, finely chopped **OPTIONAL**	.20
3 cloves of garlic, finely chopped **OPTIONAL**	.05
450g risotto rice (75g per person)	.60
Tin of chopped tomatoes	.30
2 stock cubes	.05
250g mushrooms thinly sliced	.80
1 red pepper chopped into bite size pieces (pg 15)	.40
About 30-50 pitted olives - we like green for this recipe	.30
30 cherry tomatoes, whole	£1.00
1 packet or 250g French beans, halved	£1.00
Frozen sweetcorn - about 75g **OPTIONAL**	.20
Frozen peas - about 75g **OPTIONAL**	.20
Vegan Worcester sauce (gluten free)	.10
Soy sauce (gluten free)	.05
A dash of apple cider vinegar	.05
Salt, pepper, cayenne pepper, paprika, chilli (to taste)	.10

Total £8.00 for 6 people = £1.30 each - not bad hey.

My mum used to say "watch your pennies and let the pounds do the rest"

Method

Fry or grill the sausages - until nice they are a nice light brown and crispy; put to one side.

Finely chop the onion and add to your frying pan on a medium heat with a tablespoon of oil. Meanwhile, wash, top and tail your celery then finely slice and add to the frying pan.

Cook until they are both softening up and the onion is turning a little golden brown (~10 mins). Add the garlic and cook for a further couple of minutes.

Add the rice and stir gently to coat all the grains. Add a tin of chopped tomatoes. Add the stock cube that has been dissolved in a little bit of water (use the tomato tin). Fill the empty tin with water, use that water to make sure all the rice is covered.

Add a few dashes of Worcester sauce, soy sauce and vinegar. Season with salt and pepper and a teaspoon of each of the spices.

Put the lid on the pan and now wash and slice your mushrooms and peppers - add to the pan and just stir in very gently. Make sure there is enough liquid to cover all the ingredients. Place the lid back on, bring to simmer for about 17 minutes.

This is a good time to tidy up your workstation.

Then add the cherry tomatoes and olives, stir them in very gently and put the lid back on for another 10 minutes. Pour a little more water from your tin onto the top if it's too dry. The sauce mixture wants to just cover all the ingredients.

Chop your sausages into 2cm nobbles.

Top and tail and half your French beans

Lift the lid, gently stir and taste. Add extra seasoning and water if required.

When the rice is soft, add in your peas and sweetcorn, put the French beans on top, then the sausage nobbles.

Replace the lid and steam for another 3 minutes.

Serve... a delicious healthy value midweek meal that doesn't cost you the earth.

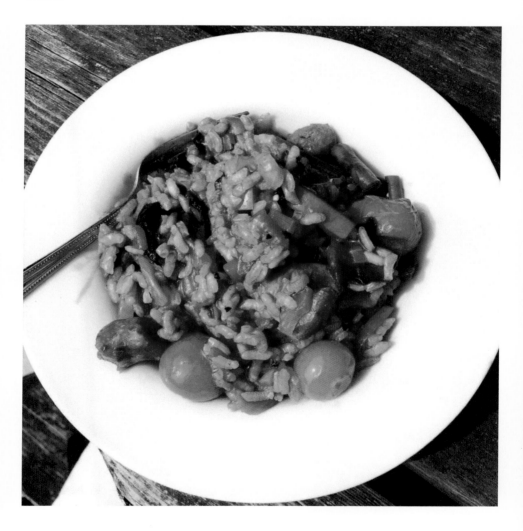

Sweet Potato Curry ✋ Ⓗ ✳

Serves 6

Ingredients

1 large onion, cut into crescent moons (like a chocolate orange)

5 cloves of garlic, finely chopped

6 cm of ginger, finely chopped

3 tsp ground cumin

4 tsp ground coriander

2 tsp cayenne pepper (add more if you like it spicier)

3 tsp paprika

5 green cardamom pods, lightly bruised

4 cloves

1.5-2 large sweet potatoes (roughly 750kg), diced into bite size cubes

2 tins of tomatoes, if you run out of tinned tomatoes, substitute 1 tin for 3 tbsp tomato puree

2 vegetable stock cubes

Dash of vegan Worcester sauce

2 tins black eyed beans, drained

9 cubes of frozen spinach

1 mug of frozen sweetcorn

2 tbsp nutritional yeast

75g cashews or 50g hulled hemp hearts

Method

Fry the onion with 2 tbsp of sunflower oil for 10 minutes, on a medium heat. Then add the garlic, ginger, cumin, coriander, cayenne pepper, cardamom and cloves and cook for a few minutes until the lovely smells are filling your kitchen.

Add in the diced sweet potato with both tins of tomatoes and enough water to cover the sweet potatoes. Bring the sauce up to a simmer and cook for 20 minutes or until the potato is cooked through, but not mushy (see if you can stick a fork in). The sweet potatoes will cook faster with the lid on; however, the sauce won't reduce so if you're in a rush make sure you don't put too much water in.

When there is about 10 minutes left on the sweet potatoes, add in the beans, spinach and sweetcorn, and continue to simmer. When the sweetcorn and beans are hot and the sweet potato is soft, your sauce is ready. Fish out the cloves and cardamom pods and serve with basmati rice (or quinoa/buckwheat if you'd like more protein), a sprinkle of nutritional yeast and the cashews/hemp hearts, for a nice crunch.

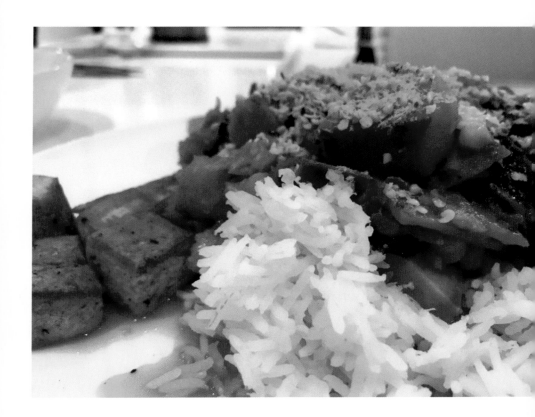

Roasted Vegetable Korma 🤚🤚 Ⓗ ❀

Ingredients

1 onion, finely diced

3 cloves of garlic, finely chopped

6 cm of ginger, finely chopped

Roasting

2 sweet potatoes, cut into bite size pieces

6 carrots, cut into 2cm slices

2 peppers, chopped

1 butternut squash, cut into bite size pieces

18 tiny button mushrooms, whole

Oil to roast

Korma Sauce

75g of cashew nuts/ sunflower seeds (pre-soak in boiled water if your blender isn't very strong)

2 tbsp sugar

1 tin of coconut milk

3 tsp cumin

3 tsp ground coriander

To start, preheat the oven to 200°C/180°C fan and chop the roasting vegetables to roughly an inch square.

Add them to a deep baking tray, coat with oil, and sprinkle on some salt and pepper. Cook for 40 minutes, or until softened. Regularly stir the tray and add additional oil if too dry.

Meanwhile, blend together all the sauce ingredients. Turn a frying pan onto medium-high heat, and start cooking the chopped onions. Once the onions have softened (after ~10 minutes), add the finely chopped ginger and garlic, and fry for roughly 5 minutes.

Once cooked, tip the roasted vegetables into the frying pan, and pour in the blended sauce. Reduce the heat on the pan and mix together all the components.

Serve on a bed of basmati rice and include some sides, such as Dad's dal (pg 140) and spinach.

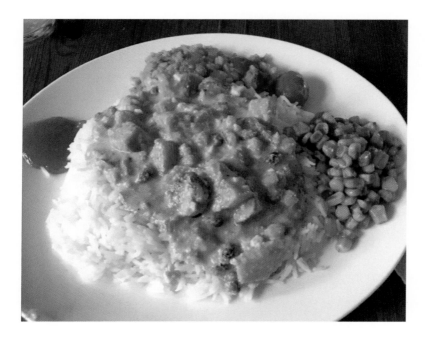

Butter Tofu ✋ Ⓗ ❀

Serves 6

This dish really does not photograph well but it's honestly one of my favourite quick dinners, so I implore you to try it because I think you'll love it too. I always try to make it in bulk, however, if I leave it out in the kitchen for even 5 minutes, all of my housemates will have tried to pilfer it, it's that good.

Ingredients

150g cashew nuts (or sunflower seeds or a tin of coconut milk can be used, however, you will have to reduce the sauce a little longer)

1 tin of tomatoes (400g)

2 stock cubes

200ml water

1½ tbsp caster sugar

1 block of firm tofu, squeezed

1 tbsp garam masala

Plenty of salt and pepper

2 tbsp cornflour

5 green cardamom pods

3 cloves

2 tsp cinnamon

Pinch of allspice **OPTIONAL** Fun fact, allspice is actually a berry!

Pinch of nutmeg **OPTIONAL**

3 large cloves of garlic, finely diced

6cm knob of ginger, finely diced

450g of dry basmati rice or 250g dry quinoa

Method

Soak the cashews in boiling water for at least an hour (I like to do this before I leave for uni in the morning).

Preheat the oven to 200°C/180°C fan.

Toss the tofu in the garam masala, salt, pepper and cornflour and place on a baking tray. Drizzle lightly with sunflower oil and cook in the oven for 20-30 minutes, turning halfway.

Drain the cashews and blend with the tomatoes, stock cubes, water and caster sugar to get a creamy sauce. Don't worry if you forgot to soak! Just add all the sauce ingredients into the pan, but with twice the amount of water and simmer for 30 mins before blending with a stick blender. Or alternatively, use coconut milk.

Heat 1 tbsp of oil in a saucepan and fry the cardamom, cloves, cinnamon, allspice, garlic and ginger over a medium-low heat for about 5 minutes until aromatic.

Add the blended sauce and bring to a simmer, simmer until it is your preferred sauce consistency. While the sauce is heating, cook the rice/quinoa according to the instructions on pg 28.

Remove the cardamom and cloves from the sauce.

I like to serve with 'easy edamames' (pg 149).

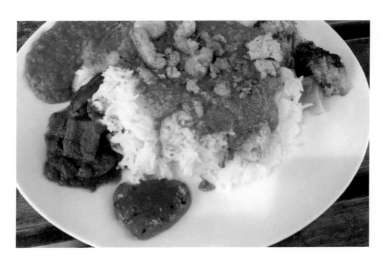

Chilli sin Carne

Serves 6

Fun fact, my favourite dinner used to be chilli con carne, with a mound of cheddar cheese, and sour cream, washed down with a pint of semi skimmed cows' milk. That's why I had very high standards for this recipe and I, personally, think that those standards are met.

Ingredients:

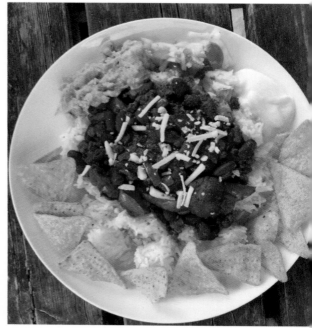

2 tbsp oil

1 onion, finely chopped

4 cloves of garlic, finely chopped

2 large tbsp of cumin

1 tbsp of coriander

1 ½ tbsp of garam marsala

1 tsp of cayenne pepper

1 cinnamon stick (or ¼ tsp more cinnamon)

½ teaspoon of cinnamon

Salt and pepper

1 fresh chilli washed and topped (I put a whole chilli per person who wants a nice spicy hot chilli and add it/put it on top of their served up chilli whole at the end) Or ½ tsp hot chilli powder

1 stock cube

1 tin of chopped tomatoes

2 large tbsp cocoa powder

1 tsp sugar

2 red peppers, chopped

300grams of button mushrooms, quartered

2 tins of kidney beans rinsed

EITHER -

1 packet of meat free mince 500g or…

3 tins of your favourite beans - turtle beans, black eye beans, black beans or….

250g brown/puy lentils, rinsed and drained.

Serve with rice, grated cheese, guacamole, salsa and tortilla crisps.

Method:

Pop the finely chopped onion and half the oil into the frying pan.

Fry for 10 minutes until soft and light brown on a medium/high heat.

Reduce the heat to medium and add the garlic. Cook for a few minutes.

Turn down the heat again, add the rest of the oil and let it heat up then...

Add the spices, salt, and pepper, and cook until you can smell the aromas. Cook for just a couple of minutes being careful not to let the spices burn, gently, slowly stirring.

Add the whole chilli.

Crumble the stock cube into the pan.

Add the tin of tomatoes + tin of water. I always rinse the tin and keep it filled with water on the side so if you need to add any extra liquid it's ready there for you to use.

Turn up the heat to bring the pan to a light boil.

Add the cocoa powder and sugar.

Add the red peppers and mushrooms and simmer for around 15 minutes.

Add the meat-free mince/beans/lentils now.

If it's too runny, take the lid off. If it's too dry, leave the lid on and add a little more water.

We like to let it simmer for 40-50 minutes to allow the lentils to cook thoroughly, however, if you're not using lentils, add the beans/ meat-free mince at the same time as the kidney beans as they take 10 around minutes.

Add the rinsed kidney beans at the end, and simmer for another 10 minutes.

During the kidney bean cooking, you can prepare your rice and accompaniments.

I recommend you add fresh chopped coriander sprinkled on top at the end to compliment the dish.

If you have any leftovers, store in the fridge until the next day or two then have as nachos, or for lunch in a wrap, or even as a filling for a jacket potato.

This whole meal costs about £6.70, per person that is £1.11.

Add the extras like fresh coriander, cheese, guacamole =

Coriander	£1.00
Cheese	£1.25 (half a pack grated)
Avocados	£1.50
Guacamole, yogurt, lime etc…	.50
Tortillas	£1.00

That brings it to a total of 11.45 divided by 6 people £1,90 per person - not bad hey for an extremely delicious and nutritious meal.

Nachos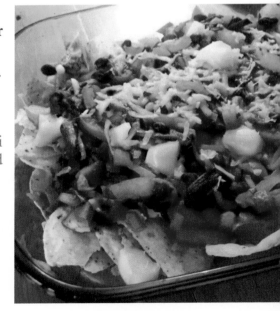

A great way to eke out last night's chilli into an extremely super quick, cheap meal.

Ingredients:

Last Night's chilli

A bag of tortilla crisps

Grated vegan cheese or my stringy cheese sauce (pg 120)

Guacamole (pg 147)

Silken tofu sour cream (pg 123)

Simple salsa (pg 147)

Pickled jalapeños

Method:

Place the crisps in an oven dish.

Spoon the chilli on top.

Grate your favourite cheese over the top.

Place under the grill on a medium heat until the cheese has melted, and the sauce is piping hot.

Add dollops of salsa, guac and sour cream.

Serve with sliced jalapenos on top.

Tuck in…

Alternatively, use the leftover chilli with some lettuce, guac, salsa and cheese to make delicious fajitas.

Theo's Fruity Curry ✋ Ⓗ ❀

This curry is perfect for students as it's uncomplicated and insanely cheap per portion.

Serves 6

450g small new potatoes

1 aubergine, cut into very thin slithers lengthways

1 onion, cut into half rings

3cm ginger, cut finely

½ a cooking apple, cut into angel wings (I like to make this on the same day I make 'Dorset apple cake' so that I can use up the apples)

3 cloves garlic, chopped finely

4 tsp curry powder

Dash soy sauce

1 pepper, cut into chunks

1 tin coconut milk

1 tin tomatoes

2 tins of beans (your choice, we use chickpeas and black-eyed beans)

Juice of ½ a lemon (roughly 1 tbsp)

To Serve

75g dry basmati rice per person

9 blocks of frozen spinach

'Dad's dal' (pg 142)

Method

Add the potatoes to a saucepan and cover with water. Add some salt and boil for roughly 15-20 minutes until soft.

While the potatoes cook, cut the aubergine into thin strips and dry fry on a medium-high heat with a sprinkle of salt. Flip the aubergine pieces after 5-6 minutes, or once the underside is lightly charred.

Once the aubergine is cooked, remove them from the pan and begin frying the onions, apple pieces and ginger, with a tbsp of oil.

After 10 minutes on a medium heat, add the garlic and curry powder and fry until fragrant (roughly 3 mins). Add a dash of soy sauce if the pan is getting dry.

Add in the rest of the ingredients and bring to a simmer.

While the sauce is cooking, cook the rice (pg 28) and the spinach, then enjoy.

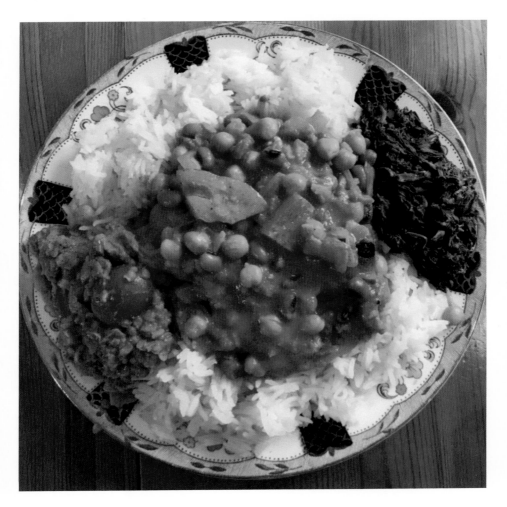

SAUCES - *Sometimes, we all just want to sauce it up a little...*

Aubergine Pasta Sauce

Makes enough for 3 portions

Wrap up **2 cloves of garlic**, with the top cut off, in tin foil. Cut the top off **1 aubergine** then cut in half lengthways. Season with salt and pepper, drizzle with olive oil and roast in the oven with the garlic for 20-30 mins at 190°C, or until really soft and tender. When they are almost finished cooking, add a whole **(250g) jar of sundried tomatoes**, with the **olive oil** into a blender, with **150g of hulled hemp hearts**, a handful of **fresh basil** and **parsley** and plenty of **salt and pepper**. Then squeeze the roasted garlic out of its skin, into the blender, add the aubergine and pulse until you have a creamy and delicious sauce. Serve with 225g of pasta of your choice.

Stringy Cheese Sauce

Enough to cover a 6-person lasagne

Blend **70g cashews (soaked)/sunflower seeds**, **1 tbsp lemon juice**, **2½ tbsp nutritional yeast**, **2 tbsp tapioca starch** (essential), **dash of soy sauce**, 2 tsp sugar, 2 tsp salt, pinch of pepper, **80ml sunflower oil**, **330ml water**, **2 tsp miso paste** (optional) and a **pinch of paprika** (optional), in a blender.

Add to a saucepan and bring to the boil gradually, stirring constantly with a whisk to ensure it doesn't stick to the bottom. After a minute or so it should've thickened up, so you can pour it into a bowl/jar and store it in the fridge until you need to use it. It will thicken as it cools.

If you can't get your hands on tapioca flour, you can use normal flour, you just won't get a stretch.

Perfect on top of vegan pizzas, nachos or stuffed into mushrooms and baked.

Classic Tomato Sauce

Enough for 6 pizzas

This is my go-to base for whenever I make pizzas.

Heat **4 tbsp olive oil** on a low heat and add 3 cloves of garlic, finely diced along with herbs of your choice (I like to use **3 tsp Italian herbs** and **2 tsp dried basil**). Cook this low and slow for about 5 minutes. Then add **1 tube of tomato puree**, **1 tbsp sugar**, plenty of **salt and pepper** and enough **water** to make it slightly runnier than your desired consistency. Simmer for 10 minutes, letting all the flavours infuse, then add a little **soy sauce**, **Worcester sauce**, **balsamic vinegar** and **lemon juice** to adjust the flavour to your liking.

If you want, you can cook some shallots on a low heat for 15 minutes at the beginning, to add more depth, however, I would then recommend blending it before spreading onto the pizzas, so it is up to you.

Raspberry Coulis

This is divine drizzled over chocolate brownie, with ice cream or with raspberry pavlova and it's mind-blowingly easy

Heat **100g of raspberries** in a small saucepan on a high heat with **2 tsp lemon juice**, crushing the raspberries with a spatula.

The sauce will start to bubble, just keep stirring until all the raspberries have become liquid.

Add **2 tbsp sugar** (you may need more, you may need less, depending on how tart you want the coulis to be) and stir in.

Taste, if it is to your liking, pour into a little serving jug to cool.

If you'd prefer it smooth, push it through a fine mesh sieve.

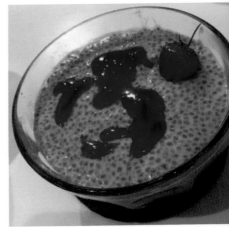

Balsamic Glaze

Heat **130ml balsamic vinegar** in a saucepan with **1 tbsp caster sugar** and a **pinch of salt** over a medium heat. Simmer for 5-10 minutes, until it thickens.

It will thicken as it cools so a good way to test if it is thick enough is to take a teaspoon of it and spread it on a plate in the fridge so that it cools quickly, then you can see if it is the consistency you'd like.

Beware, don't breathe in the steam as it is pretty potent so will make your eyes water.

Mint Yoghurt Dressing

Mix together **200g dairy free yoghurt** (we like to use Alpro Plain) with **1½ tbsp mint sauce** (can add more/less depending on how minty you like it). Then season with **salt and pepper** and garnish with fresh coriander/parsley depending on the dish.

Tahini Dressing

Tahini is naturally a little bitter so if that isn't to your taste, add more sugar.

Mix together (using a balloon whisk helps here) **6 tbsp tahini, 4 tbsp water, 4 tsp oil, 3-4 tbsp lemon juice** (or to taste), **3 pinches of sugar, salt, pepper,** and a **large pinch of paprika** (optional).

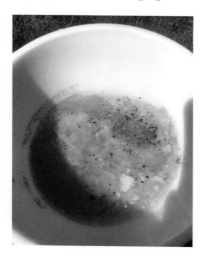
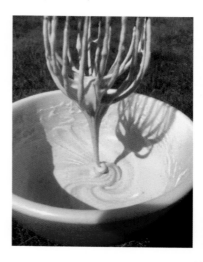

Salad Dressing

Mix together 2 tbsp apple cider vinegar, 2 tbsp extra virgin olive oil, 1 tsp honey, 1 tbsp Balsamic Vinegar, ½ a lime squeezed, 2 tsp Wholegrain Mustard.

Silken Tofu Sour Cream

Blend together **1 block of silken tofu (349g)** with **2 tbsp lime juice, 2 tbsp sunflower oil, 2 tsp apple cider vinegar,** 2½ tsp sugar and season with **salt** to taste.

With Sundried Tomatoes:

+1 tbsp lime, 6 sundried tomatoes, sprinkle of cayenne pepper

With Fresh Herbs:

+1 tbsp lime, fresh mint/coriander/parsley/chives/any fresh herbs you might like

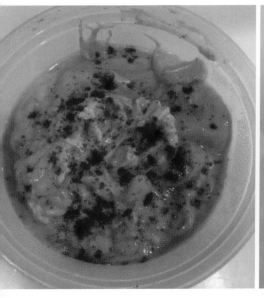 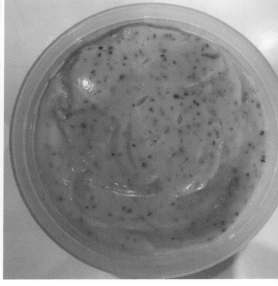

SATURDAYS AND SUNDAYS - *Recipes that are a little more unusual, perfect to make with family and friends on the weekends.*

Sushi with Watermelon 'Tuna'

This made enough for 6 people to each do one roll, however, it isn't overly filling, so you could double the recipe if you think that wouldn't be enough. If you don't like sushi, make the tuna and have it with rice and avocados, like a poke bowl. **Warning: you do have to marinade the watermelon overnight, so make sure you plan ahead.**

Ingredients

For the 'tuna'
One large watermelon

For the Marinade
240ml water
150ml soy sauce I know it seems like a lot, but you can reuse this marinade
3 tbsp capers
2 tbsp brine (either from olives or capers)
100ml sunflower oil
3 tsp smoked paprika
1 tsp paprika
3 tsp garlic powder or roughly 5 cloves
Plenty of salt
2 nori sheets (unless you're making it into sushi then 1 should suffice)
Juice of 1 lemon
4 tbsp sriracha or other spicy sauce (optional)

For the Sushi

You can do any fillings you want really, but I'll list the ones we like to do

2 carrots, sliced into thin slithers (using a peeler helps)

12cm cucumber, cut into strips

3 spring onions, cut into strips

2 avocados, sliced (pg 18)

1 red pepper, cut into strips (pg 16)

100g tenderstem broccoli, cut in half lengthways

Wasabi paste **OPTIONAL**

6 sheets of nori (we would recommend getting 2 packs of Yukata Sushi Nori for this whole dish)

For the Rice

250g sushi rice

1 tbsp mirin

2 tbsp cooking sake

2 tbsp caster sugar

1 tbsp salt

Method

1) Cut the top and bottom off the watermelon then cut off the green skin.

2) Then, place it on its side, with the sliced top on the right and the sliced bottom on the left.

3) Then slice in 3cm intervals. You should essentially end up with big coins that have the diameter of your watermelon and a depth of 3 cm.

4) Cut these coins into 3 triangles by making 2 diagonal cuts across the face of each coin (don't worry if these are quite big, they will shrink when cooked).

5) Then put these 'fillets' into a large bowl. If you can be bothered, you can remove the seeds for a more realistic texture, but I never do.

(See next page for diagram).

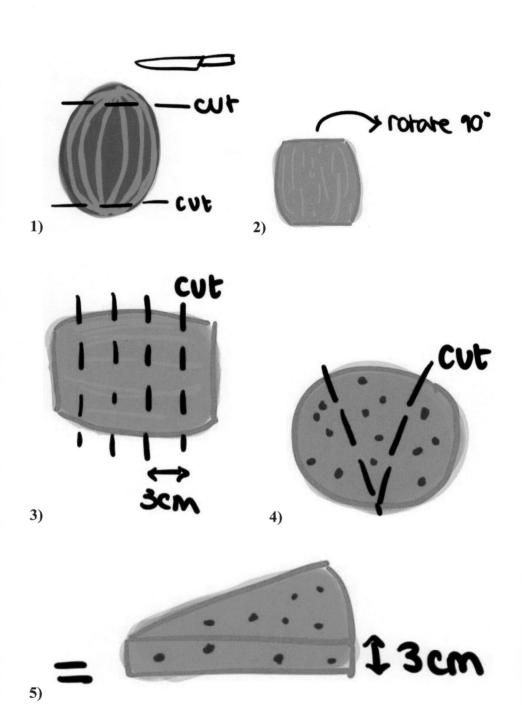

1)

2) rotate 90°

3) 3cm

4) cut

5) = ↕3cm

126

Now it is time to make the marinade. Add all of the other 'tuna' ingredients into a blender/food processor and blend on high speed until the nori and the capers are in small pieces.

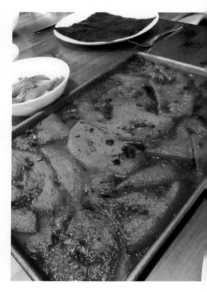

Then pour this sauce into the bowl/s with the watermelon in and leave to marinade overnight.

On the next day, place the watermelon fillets onto a baking tray, spoon on some of the marinade and bake at 200°C fan for 40 minutes to 1 hour, or until soft. When cooked they will have the consistency of raw tuna.

Top tip: cover the tray with tin foil to help keep your oven clean.

While the 'tuna' is cooking, cook the sushi rice according to the instructions on the packet.

It will say this on the packet, but the key with sushi rice is to rinse it very thoroughly and then rinse again. Starchy rice is the enemy here.

Mix together the sake, mirin, sugar and salt in a small bowl, ready to mix with the rice once cooked.

While the rice is cooking, I like to cut up the veg that I'm using and cook the broccoli and peppers. I cook them in a dry frying pan, on a high heat for 5-10 minutes, or long enough to char them.

This is a good time to clear the workstation.

Hopefully everything should be cooked at this point. If you want, you can cool it all before rolling the sushi, but we rarely bother as we are always too impatient.

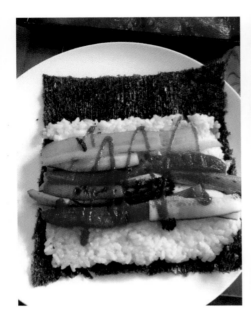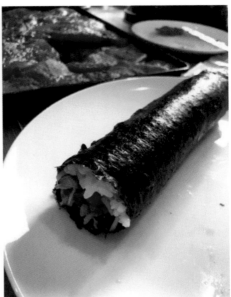

The next steps in the method are on the nori packaging so you can read that instead if you like, but I'm summarising here:

Place your nori sheet on a **dry** plate.

Spread your rice ⅔rds of the way up your nori sheet.

Make an indent in the middle of your rice and add in whatever toppings you'd like. I thinly sliced the 'tuna' fillets so they would go in the sushi better.

Using slightly damp hands, roll from the bottom up, then slice into bite size pieces using a *very sharp*, wet knife.

We don't have a bamboo rolling mat as many methods suggest and it works fine, just make sure that you roll tightly.

Enjoy with some soy sauce, wasabi or any other sauces that you'd like.

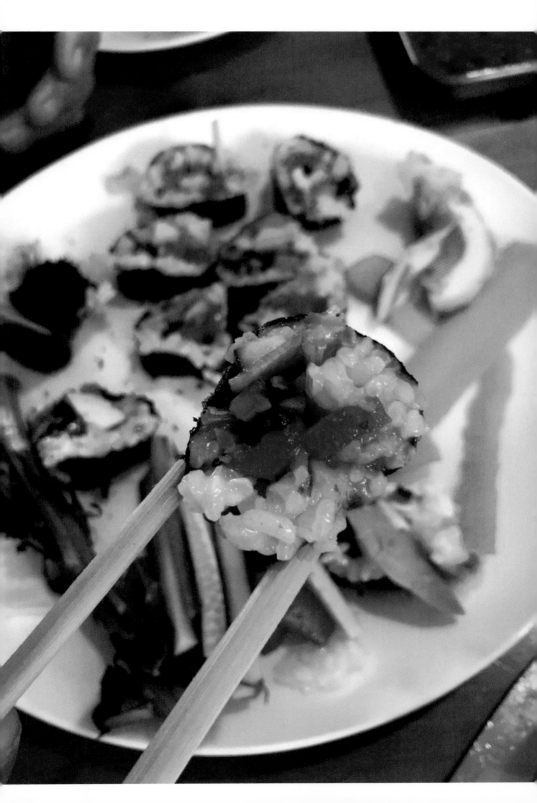

Pizzas

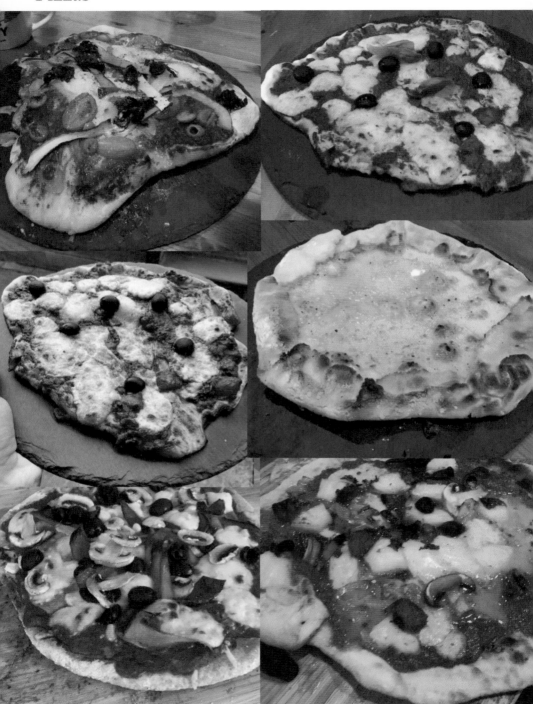

For the Base

You could use –

- **Tortilla wraps**
- **Shop bought bases**

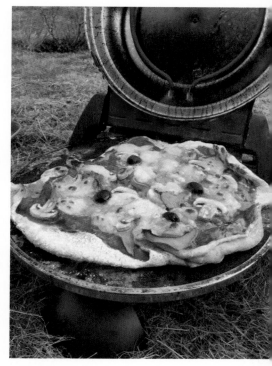

Alternatively, you can make your own dough:

- **Homemade pizza dough** *(enough for 2 pizzas)*

Fill a bowl with 300g strong white flour.

Put ½ tsp yeast on one side of the bowl with ½ tsp sugar.

Put 1 tsp of salt on the other side of the bowl.

Add 160ml of water and 1 tbsp of olive oil gradually while kneading (either by hand or with a mixer with a dough hook), until smooth and stretchy.
Add more water if it is too dry, add more flour if it's too sticky.

Leave in a bowl, with cling film on top, in a warm place for 45 minutes to 1 hour to prove.

Then roll it out with a little semolina/flour and enjoy.

- **Homemade gluten free dough**- inspired by Doves Farm Gluten free white bread flour (*2 pizzas*):

Mix 10g chickpea flour with 140ml water (or you can make ½ a flax egg, page 27), 1½ tbsp oil, ½ tsp vinegar, 1 tbsp sugar and ½ tsp salt with a whisk.

Add in 250g of gf strong white flour and 1 tsp quick yeast and knead, adding more water/flour to get the right consistency.

Leave in a cling film covered bowl for 45 mins to 1 hour to prove.

Roll out and enjoy.

For the Toppings

- **Margherita** - 'classic tomato sauce, (pg 121) with either shop bought vegan mozzarella, or homemade "stringy cheese sauce" (pg 120).
- **Pepperoni** - 'classic tomato sauce' with cheese and your favourite vegan chorizo replacement (we like "shroomdogs"), cut into slices and fried.
- **Hawaiian** - 'classic tomato sauce', vegan ham of choice (we like "Quorn ham free slices"), mushrooms and pineapple.
- **Sweet chilli 'chicken'** - 'classic tomato sauce', vegan chicken of choice or 'crispy tofu pieces' (pg 152), favourite vegan sweet chilli sauce (we like Blue Dragon) and thin slices of red pepper.
- **Texas BBQ** - BBQ sauce base, caramelised red onions (pg 148), thinly sliced red and green peppers, sweetcorn and vegan chicken of choice or 'crispy tofu pieces'.
- **Veggie Medley** - 'classic tomato sauce' base, thin slithers of courgette, sun dried tomatoes, sweetcorn and fresh rocket at the end.
- **Taste of the Sea** - classic tomato base, crushed capers, sliced garlic cloves, green and black olives and thin slices of large flat mushrooms with the stalk taken out to look like anchovies.
- **Bechamel Base** - use the bechamel sauce recipe (pg 62) as the base, then add vegan ham slices, sliced mushrooms, garlic vegan butter and plenty of vegan mozzarella.

Cooking

- If you're using a tortilla wrap, grill under a high heat for 2-4 minutes. Don't over-sauce your wrap or you'll end up with a soggy pizza.

- If you're using a bought base/homemade base, cook in the oven, on a lined tray, at around 200°C fan for 10 - 15 minutes, you're looking for the base to be cooked through and the cheese to be lovely and melted. The dough may take longer to cook if you have rolled it out quite thickly so make sure you give the crust a poke before you take it out of the oven and if it doesn't spring back then the inside is raw.

- If you have a pizza stone and are making your own base, set the oven to the highest heat possible and preheat the pizza stone. Then move the pizza onto the stone and cook for 5 minutes or less on the top shelf of your oven. Having a pizza stone helps to make a really crisp base and being at the top of the oven cooks the top of the pizza in that time. Make sure you have thoroughly floured/semolina-ed the bottom of your pizza base when you put it onto the stone, or it will get stuck which will be very stressful.

- If you have a portable pizza oven, like in the picture on pg 131, it is almost the same as the pizza stone, just preheat it and cook your pizzas for 4-5 minutes.

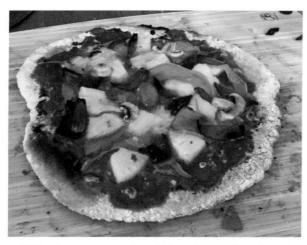

(This is an example of the gluten free base)

Sweet and Sour Tofu

Serves 6

You will never want to go to the takeaway again once you have tried this.

Ingredients

1 batch of 'crispy tofu pieces' (pg 152)

1 tablespoon of oil

2 onions, roughly chopped

Salt, pepper and 1 teaspoon of sugar

4 cloves of garlic, finely chopped

A large knobble of ginger, finely chopped

100-150grams of cashew nuts **OPTIONAL**

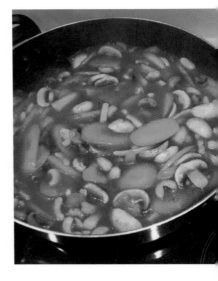

A few drops of sesame oil

1 tsp cayenne pepper

1 tbsp paprika

A pinch of chilli

½ tsp cinnamon

1 tbsp honey

A dash of each - cooking sake, mirin, soy sauce and Worcester sauce (gluten free if necessary)

1 pack of baby corn, broken in half

5 carrots, sliced at an angle

250g button mushrooms, sliced or halved if they are small

300ml of pineapple or orange juice

A pineapple or a tin of pineapple rings, cut into 8ths

1 tin of water chestnuts

1 tin of bamboo shoots

For the Sauce

2 tbsp cornflour

2 tbsp soy sauce gluten free

5 tbsp cider vinegar

1 tbsp tomato ketchup

1 tbsp brown sugar

To Serve

1 leafy green cabbage - sweetheart, savoy, pointed white

1 mug of frozen peas (around 150g)

75g dried basmati per person

Method

Prepare 1 portion of crispy fried tofu, put to one side. Then put 1 tbsp of oil and half of the finely chopped onions in the frying pan. On a medium heat sauté, them for 10 minutes or until golden brown.

Season with salt and brown sugar, then add the ginger and garlic. Sauté for another 5 minutes until the ginger is soft and well cooked.

Push the onions, ginger and garlic to the side and pour the cashew nuts into the middle of your pan. Make sure each cashew nut is flat/touching the base of the pan so that they brown on one side.... leave for about 4 minutes to brown, then flip them over to brown on the other side.

Add a few drops of sesame oil, then stir in the cayenne pepper, paprika, dried chilli, cinnamon, honey, sake, mirin, soy sauce and Worcester sauce.

Add the halved baby corn, sliced carrots, mushrooms and other half of the finely chopped onions to the pan. Add the orange juice, bring almost to the boil, then simmer with the lid on for 15-20 minutes. Add more juice if the vegetables aren't covered.

Meanwhile prepare your cabbage: - shred the cabbage, add to a microwaveable dish, add salt, pepper, a knobble of flora, throw in the frozen peas, cover and microwave for about 4 minutes depending on your microwave. Put these to one side to warm for a further couple of minutes just before serving.

Get your rice on the go, clear your workstation and get ready to make the sauce.

In a mug/jug put 2 large tablespoons of cornflour add a little water and mix making sure all the powder is mixed in with the water. Put to one side.

Going back to your frying pan, check that the carrots are cooked. When they are al dente (have a slight bite), add the pineapple slices, bamboo shoots and water chestnuts. Add 2 tablespoons soy sauce, 5 tablespoons cider vinegar, 1 tablespoon tomato ketchup, 1 tablespoon brown sugar. Add more seasoning now, if necessary. You may not need this much brown sugar, it depends on the sweetness of the juice you use, so add a little at first, then taste.

Now for the finale - give the cornflour a little stir to make sure all the flour has mixed in, add it to your frying pan and as it heats up it should thicken up. If it isn't thick enough, make up a little more corn flour with water; or if it's too thick add some more juice to the pan.

Then while the sauce is thickening add the tofu. Or if you like the tofu to remain crispy put it on the top once you have served. Enjoy with the cabbage, peas and cooked basmati rice.

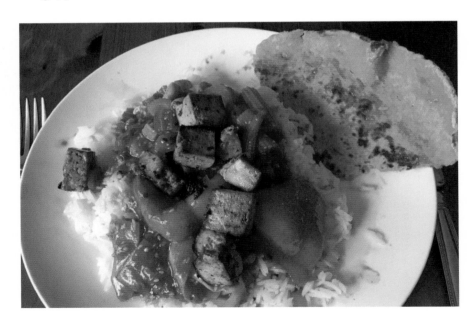

Foley Bean Burger

Makes 15 burgers with the dehydrated soy protein, probably about 10 without.

Ingredients

2 tins of beans, drained and rinsed (we use black beans and black eyed, however, using all black will result in a meatier looking burger)

200g cashews (could replace with sunflower seeds/ more breadcrumbs)

2 flax 'eggs'

1 onion, cut into fine half rings, it is important that you cut them like this as they make tendrils in the burger which help keep it together.

1 pepper, finely chopped (we put ours in the food processor, but you don't have to)

4 cloves garlic, finely diced

6 sundried tomatoes, blended/finely chopped

1 tsp cayenne pepper (add more to taste)

2 tsp smoked paprika

2 tsp normal paprika

2 tsp sugar

1½ tsp salt

10 grinds pepper

2 tbsp of sunflower oil

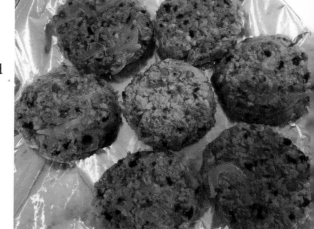

100g dehydrated soy protein, rehydrated and squeezed **OPTIONAL**

1 tbsp tapioca starch or 75g breadcrumbs/crushed cornflakes, tapioca starch is ideal here as it is like glue, holding the burger together, however, as far as I know, you can only get it online so if you don't have any, feel free to use breadcrumbs to absorb moisture, it won't be the same but it will still be delicious.

100g dairy-free cheese of choice (I like it with mozzarella or a smoky flavoured cheese)

2 tbsp vegan mayonnaise

A dash of Worcester sauce

Method

Preheat the oven to 200°C/180°C fan.

Pour the beans onto a tray and put in the oven for 20 minutes to dry out.

Add the cashews to another baking tray and roast in the oven for around 10 minutes, or until lightly browned.

Make the flax eggs by combining 2 tbsp flax seeds (no need to finely blend for this recipe) with 6 tbsp water and refrigerating for 15 minutes.

While the beans and cashews are in the oven, fry the onion, pepper, garlic, spices, salt and pepper, in 2 tbsp of oil, on a medium heat for around 10 minutes.

Rehydrate the soy protein according to the instructions on the package.

Pour the cooked onions and pepper into a bowl, while still hot, and add the tapioca starch/breadcrumbs and stir to thoroughly mix.

When the beans and cashews are finished baking, allow them to cool for a few minutes, until pouring into the food processor with the cheese, blitz a few times until the cashews are finely chopped. If you don't have a food processor, you can do this by hand.

Squeeze out as much water as you can from the rehydrated protein and add to the onions, along with the bean and cashew mix.

Add the mayo and Worcester sauce and mix until thoroughly incorporated.

Use your hands to form patties and place on a lined baking tray.

Put the baking tray in the fridge/freezer for 15 minutes to firm up then cook as desired.

For baking (my preferred method):

Bake at 180°C fan for 20-30 mins, flipping halfway through. If you want to you can then put them under the grill for an extra 3 minutes on either side, just to crisp up the outside.

For frying:

Drizzle some sunflower oil into the frying pan (enough to cover the bottom) and heat to a medium-high temperature.

Fry for 6 minutes on either side, or until crispy and delicious.

Serve with caramelised red onions (pg 148), sliced lettuce, thin slices of tomato and toasted bread buns.

If you can't eat them all at once, freeze them after cooking so when you just want a quick dinner, all you have to do is bung it in the oven.

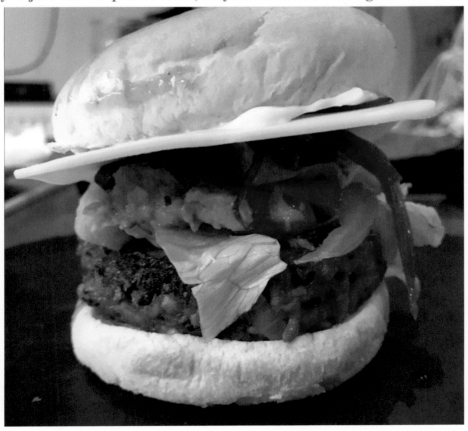

SIDES - *If you think that the main isn't going to fill you up, then why not make a super side, or to put it another way, it just means that you can eke out your main and have enough for leftovers another day.*

Roasted Sweet Potatoes

This is probably the tastiest, healthiest and easiest side that you can make. They are super quick and easy, richer in nutrients and lower GI than normal potatoes. Throw those oven chips in the bin and get some of these delicious treats on the go.

You will develop your own "perfect" way of cooking them and a bit of care goes a long way in getting exactly what you want. But here is how I do them:

Ingredients

I use about ½ large sweet potato per person, as a side

Sweet potatoes

Cooking oil (we use sunflower)

Salt pepper

Paprika **OPTIONAL**

Method

Preheat the oven to 220°C/200°C fan.

The way that you cut the potatoes is important. Too large and they will not be fluffy in the middle. Too small and they will dry out. I go for one-inch squares. This is about 2.5 cm.

Put them into a baking tray. Pour on a glug of oil. Dose liberally with freshly ground salt and pepper and mix it all up with your fingers. Sprinkle over some paprika.

Once the oven is hot, pop then in. Turn them all over after 20 minutes with a spatula.

Remove from the oven after half an hour total. They should be sweet, slightly brown and caramelised one the edges and soft and fluffy in the middle.

Serve straight from the oven. Yum.

Tip. If you are cooking a lot, spread it over a couple of trays. If you pile them up on the tray they won't crisp properly.

Tip 2. Don't bother taking the skin off the sweet potatoes, just wash thoroughly.

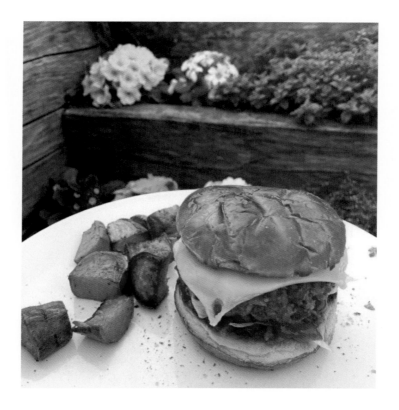

Dad's Dal

Serves 10

I always used to think that dal is that dreadful runny substance that you order once from the curry house and never try again. Fear not. With a bit of attention, you can produce this thick and delicious side dish that really enhances any curry and can be eaten on its own as a hearty winter warmer. Once you have the knack it's really easy.

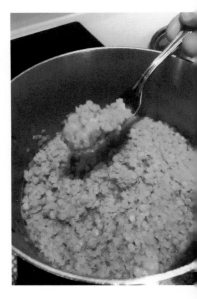

Ingredients

1 mug red lentils (roughly 200g)

1 level tsp turmeric

Knob of vegan butter

A boiled kettle - I use about 2 mugs of water (roughly 560ml) to one cup of lentils

A generous glug of sunflower oil

1 onion, finely diced

Thumb of ginger, finely diced

1 garlic clove, finely diced

A chilli, if you're feeling spicy, sliced

1 heaped tsp cumin

1 heaped tsp coriander

1 heaped tsp garam masala

2 large handfuls of cherry tomatoes, whole

2 blocks frozen spinach per person **OPTIONAL**

Method

This does take a little bit of attention to get the best results. Ideally you are looking for a thick luscious dal where you can still make out the individual lentils, so it is not a soup. The lentils should be soft but not mushy. The keys to this are adding the water slowly as it cooks and stirring gently and infrequently - just enough to make sure it doesn't stick, without breaking up the lentils.

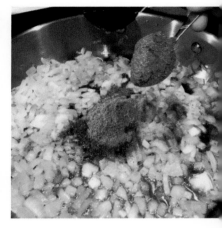

Boil the kettle so that the hot water is ready.

Rinse the lentils thoroughly in a sieve.

Add lentils to a medium saucepan with enough boiling water to *just* cover them, along with the spread and turmeric.

Bring to a gentle simmer. Stir gently with a fork every 3 to 4 minutes.

Top up slowly with the boiled water as it is absorbed to ensure that the lentils are only just covered.

Don't add any more water after 15 minutes, use the last 5 minutes to let the water evaporate and absorb so that about half of the lentils are covered.

After 20 minutes in total, turn off and cover with a lid.

Next make the flavouring. You can do what you like here but I use a simple tarka recipe. If you are in a hurry you can always make this while the lentils are cooking.

Gently fry the finely chopped onions, ginger and chilli, in a frying pan, on a medium heat for about 10 minutes, stirring occasionally to ensure nothing burns. Don't be afraid to use plenty of oil (around 2 tbsp) as the spices need to cook in the oil.

Once they are cooked nicely add the ginger and spices and stir to ensure that everything is coated in a spicy, oily mix.

Add the tomatoes and cook gently for a further 5-10 minutes until the first tomato starts to split, again stirring occasionally. The tomatoes should remain largely whole as they will pack a flavour punch and don't want to be mashed up into the mix.

Pour the lentils into the spice mixture and add the spinach, if using.

Stir gently to mix it all together without mashing up the lentils and cook at a very low heat for 5 minutes being careful not to let it stick.

Ideally serve with a blob of vegan yoghurt and some chopped coriander - delicious.

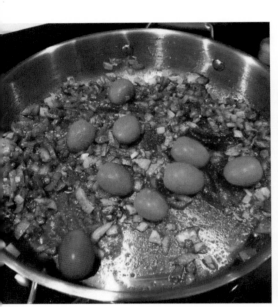
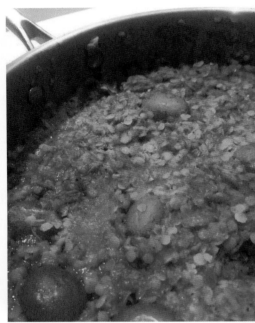

Auntie Shoba's Dal

Serves 10

Ingredients

300g chana dal (dried split chickpeas)

2 tbsp dried cumin

1 tsp turmeric

1 clove of garlic, diced

1cm ginger, diced

1 green chilli, cut in half

350ml water/ enough water to cover the chickpeas

1 large carrot, diced

1/3 coconut block with hot water to make 1 cup coconut milk, alternatively, you can use half a tin of coconut milk

1 tbsp tamarind paste/ lemon juice, you can adjust this to suit your own taste, depending on how tangy you want it to be.

10 blocks frozen spinach

1 tbsp mustard seeds

1 white onion, finely sliced

1 tsp dried chilli flakes **OPTIONAL**

Method

Put the chana dal, cumin, turmeric, garlic, ginger, chilli and water into a saucepan and bring to a simmer.

Simmer for 30 minutes then add the diced carrot and simmer until the chickpeas can be crushed between 2 fingers (up to another 10 minutes).

Regularly check that there is sufficient water so that nothing sticks.

Add the coconut milk, tamarind/ lemon juice and frozen spinach, stir and keep warm while you do the next step.

In a separate, dry frying pan, fry the mustard seeds until they start to pop, then add the sliced onions and chilli flakes, with 1 tbsp sunflower oil and fry for 10 minutes, or until the onion is golden.

Toss this in with the chickpea mix, season to taste and enjoy.

OPTIONAL, serve with a sprinkle of fresh coriander leaves.

My Take on Bruschetta

Serves 1

This is really easy and looks really fancy as a starter for a meal or even just as a snack. It is essentially bruschetta but deconstructed, and the tomatoes are cooked.

Ingredients

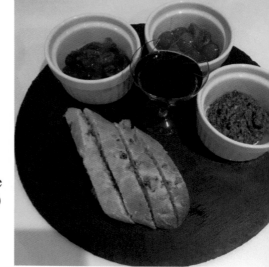

60g cherry tomatoes

Sprinkle of salt

Sprinkle of sugar

Sprinkle of pepper

20ml olive oil

20ml balsamic vinegar

Bake at home bread of choice (I like the Tesco 'bake at home petit pain')

Tapenade (pg 158)

Caramelised red onions (pg 148)

Method

Preheat the oven to 180°C/160°C fan.

Half the cherry tomatoes and season the face with the sugar, salt and pepper.

Then, place them face down on a baking tray, with a drizzle of olive oil and balsamic vinegar.

Bake for 15-20 minutes until soft and sweet.

Meanwhile, cook your bake at home bread according to the packaging and cook the red onions, if having.

While the cherry tomatoes are baking, put the tapenade and onions into a ramekin (if you want to look fancy) and pour the oil and balsamic vinegar into a little bowl for dipping the bread into.

When the tomatoes are done put them into a ramekin too (optional) and enjoy while hot.

This dish is easy to scale if you're having it as a family, just keep the onions and tomatoes in their baking trays and bring a spatula to the table so people can just help themselves.

Simple Salsa

Serves 5

120g cherry tomatoes, quartered

1 small onion, finely diced

3 large pinches sugar

Salt and pepper

6 tsp apple cider vinegar

Handful of fresh coriander, roughly chopped (optional)

1 hot chilli, finely sliced (optional)

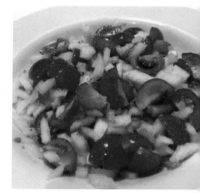

Guacamole

Serves 6

4 avocados (pg 18)

2 tbsp dairy-free yoghurt

1 lime, juiced (~2 tbsp)

2 tsp dairy-free cream (e.g. Alpro Single Soya) **OPTIONAL**

Salt and Pepper

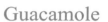

Slice the avocados lengthways around the entire oval. Twist the two halves to take them apart. Use a spoon to lever out the stones. Place one of the stones in the guacamole bowl - This will preserve the vibrant green colour of the avocado!

Add the yoghurt, cream and lime juice. Then, mash together all the ingredients with a utensil of choice (I prefer a spoon. You may use a fork...). Once the guacamole is smooth, add salt and pepper to taste. Top Tip: The salt draws out the delicious flavours but remember to not overpower the freshness of the lime.

Minted Peas

Serves 6

Ingredients

3 mugs, roughly 450g, of frozen peas (my mum swears by Birdseye)

2 tbsp extra virgin olive oil

Lots of salt and pepper

1 bunch of fresh mint, de-stalked, washed and roughly chopped

Method

Put the peas into a large bowl and cover with boiling water. Let stand for a few minutes then drain. By cooking them this way, it stops any risk of them overcooking and going mushy.

Put the peas back into the bowl and add the other ingredients. Microwave for 1-2 minutes to ensure the peas are piping hot. Toss the peas to ensure they're thoroughly coated and enjoy while hot.

Caramelised Red Onion

Serves 6, however, we always want more

Ingredients

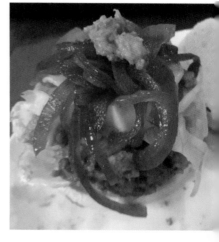

2 red onions, chopped into rings (pg 14)

2 tsp sugar

2 tsp salt

2 tbsp balsamic vinegar

1-2 tbsp neutral cooking oil

Method

To begin, chop the red onions in half lengthways, remove the skin and slice finely into half rings. Add the onions to a small tray/frying pan, then coat in the sugar, salt, vinegar, and oil.

Method 1) Fry the onions on the hob at a medium-high heat for roughly 15 minutes.

Method 2) Cook the onion in the oven on 200°C/180°C for 15-20 minutes. The caramelisation is complete when the onions are soft and have a crispy brown coating.

Easy Peasy Edamames

Serves 6

One of my friends recommended edamame beans to me in 1st year so I excitedly bought some on my next Tesco delivery. They are a complete protein source, high in vitamins and minerals and have links to reducing certain types of cancer, sounds amazing right!? Unfortunately, I did not know that you had to suck them out of their pods, so I spent weeks cooking them in all different ways only to result in the same leathery, inedible pod. Luckily, I have now learnt that lesson so I can now pass it onto you, saving you lots of time and confusion!

Ingredients

450g frozen edamame beans (75g per person)

2 tbsp extra virgin olive oil

Lots of salt and pepper

2 fresh chillies, sliced (optional)

Method

When I'm at uni, because I'm lazy, I like to cook my rice, serve it, and then quickly cook the edamames in the same pan so that I don't have to wash the rice out, but I probably wouldn't advise that.

Place the edamame beans into a pan of boiling water and simmer for 5-6 minutes, covered.

Drain the beans then put back into the pan and add the oil, salt, pepper and fresh chillies.

Toss the beans to ensure they're coated then serve.

Eat by placing the top of the pod into your mouth and squeezing the bottom until one of the beans pops out. This means you can enjoy all the flavouring that you tossed the pods in.

Sometimes the edamame beans you get in supermarkets are already shelled, you can prepare those in the same way

Toasted Cashews

Allow around 12g cashews per person for sprinkling on top of a meal.

Preheat the oven to around 200°C/180°C fan and dry roast for 8-10 minutes, or until golden brown.

Tempeh

Makes enough for 12-16 portions, we like to freeze half.

This is one of the easiest things to make. It can be used and cooked in the same way as tofu and provides a nice firm texture which can make a nice change. The only reason we don't use tempeh more in this cookbook is because it is often more difficult to find in supermarkets than tofu.

Both are soy products, low in sodium and free from cholesterol. Tempeh provides more protein, fibre, iron and potassium whereas tofu contains more calcium and is lower in calories. Also, making your own means less plastic is used.

Ingredients

2 mugs dry soybeans (400g)

4 tbsp cider vinegar

¾ tsp tempeh starter (easily purchased online)

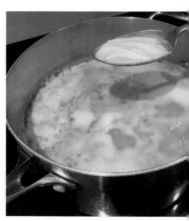

Method

Soak the beans overnight in plenty of water

Drain and rinse the beans

Put the beans in a large saucepan and fill with water to one inch above the beans

Bring to the boil with the lid off and simmer for 50 minutes

You will notice a foam appearing on top - skim that off with a spoon

Stir from time to time to ensure that it does not stick

Next add the cider vinegar and cook for a further 20 minutes until the water has nearly all disappeared

The beans should now be whole but soft and easily crushed

Drain any remaining water

Leave to cool to 35 °C - should feel warm but not hot to the touch

Add the tempeh starter and mix well

Use a masher to break the beans up a bit. You don't want mash, but you don't want it to be basically just beans - somewhere in between gives the best texture

Put the mixture into a plastic bag doubled over to prevent leakage and make one-inch spaced holes in the bag with a cocktail stick to allow the air in. It should be fairly well packed in.

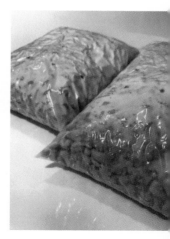

Store in a warm spot such as an airing cupboard, proving drawer. I put it on top of a cupboard near the boiler. Too hot will kill it so it must be around 35 degrees.

Leave for 48 hours

When it looks white and stuck together then your tempeh is ready.

This can be frozen if not required at present.

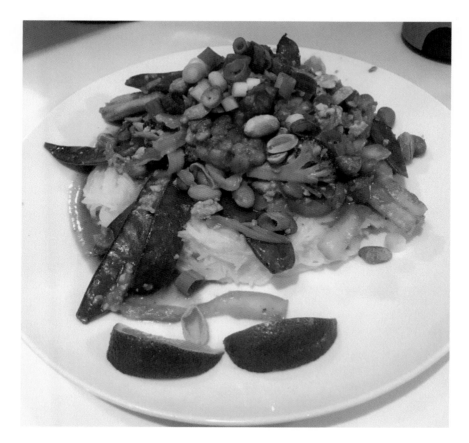

Crispy Tofu Pieces

Serves 6

If I have the oven on for a recipe, I will cook the tofu in the oven as per Method 1, otherwise I will just use Method 2.

Ingredients

1 block of firm tofu, squeezed (pg 22)

2 tbsp cornflour

2 tsp paprika

1 tsp garlic powder (optional)

Generous sprinkle of salt and pepper

Drizzle of sunflower oil

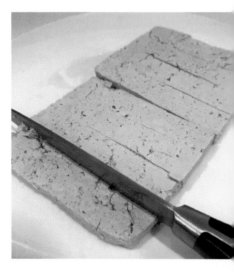

Method 1

Squeeze the tofu, as shown on pg 22.

Preheat the oven to 200°C/180°C fan.

Cut the block into bite size pieces. If using Cauldron tofu, cut in half widthways, and then quarters in both directions, to make cubes.

Put the tofu pieces into a bowl and add the cornflour, paprika, garlic powder, salt and pepper. Toss the pieces until they're covered then transfer to a non-stick/lined baking tray (shaking off any excess flour).

Drizzle the tofu pieces with the sunflower oil and bake for 30 minutes, or until crispy. Don't forget to turn halfway.

Enjoy while still hot.

Method 2

Squeeze the tofu, as shown on page 22.

Heat up 1-2 tbsp sunflower oil in a large saucepan, on a medium heat, if you have a small saucepan or a weaker stove, it is good to do it in 2 batches, so in that case add 1 tbsp per batch.

Put the tofu pieces into a bowl and add the cornflour, paprika, garlic powder, salt and pepper.

Toss the pieces until they're covered then transfer to the frying pan, the oil should sizzle when the tofu is added. Fry for 7-10 minutes on either side, or until golden brown.

Enjoy while still hot, sprinkled over a meal, or just as a snack.

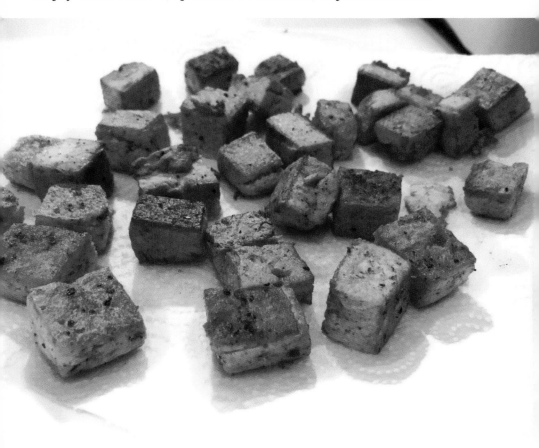

Miso Glazed Aubergines

Serves 2

Ingredients

1 aubergine, washed and sliced in half lengthways (no need to remove the stalk)

2 tbsp soy sauce

2 tbsp mirin

2 tbsp miso paste

1 tbsp sugar

1 tbsp sunflower oil

Method

Preheat the oven to 180°C/160°C fan.

Cross hatch the faces of the aubergine halves.

Heat a non-stick frying pan on a high heat and place the aubergine halves face down. Cook for 10 minutes face down then flip and cook for 5 minutes skin side down. You don't want the heat to be so high that the aubergines are burning, but a little char is okay.

While the aubergine is cooking, mix together all the other ingredients in a little bowl.

By this point, the aubergines should be soft to touch (i.e. your finger leaves an indent).

Take the aubergines off the heat and gently pour the sauce into the cross hatches. Place the aubergines on a lined baking tray and cover with tin foil.

Bake in the oven for 30-45 minutes, or until the inside of the aubergine is soft and delicious.

Enjoy.

Cauliflower Cheese

Serves 6

Ingredients

1 large cauliflower

My stringy cheese sauce (pg 120)

You can make the stringy cheese sauce with normal cornflour in this recipe, if you don't have any tapioca starch.

100ml unsweetened plant milk (this is just to give the desired consistency; you may not need the whole amount)

1 tbsp vegan single cream (I like Alpro Single Soya)

Method

Prepare and cook the cauliflower as on pg 19.

While the cauliflower is in the microwave, cook the cheesy sauce until thick and stretchy.

Pour the sauce, cream and a little milk into the cauliflower bowl, mix well and place back into the microwave for a few minutes so that the cauliflower can soak up the sauce.

Use a spoon to break the cauliflower into large florets and enjoy.

I like this with a nut roast or a really spicy curry.

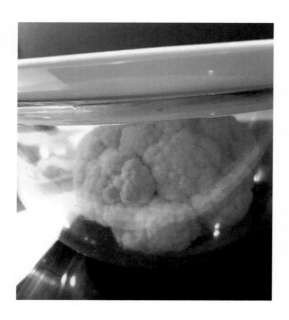

SNACKS - *Fancy a tasty, healthy, kind to you and the planet snack?*

Hummus

Ingredients

2 tins of chickpeas

4 cloves of garlic crushed

1 tbsp olive oil

1 tbsp sunflower oil

1 tbsp tahini

1 tsp caster sugar

Salt and pepper

200-300 ml *cold* water

Sprinkle of peri peri salt **OPTIONAL**

Method

There are two key components to this recipe that make it superior to other hummus recipes you have tried in the past.

1) You boil the chickpeas which softens them, resulting in a much creamier texture.

2) You crush the garlic and let it sit while the chickpeas are boiling.

One thing I really don't like about homemade hummus' in the past is that bitter raw garlic aftertaste that often accompanies it. By crushing your garlic and allowing it to sit, this is eliminated.

Simmer chickpeas for 20-30mins

While the chickpeas are simmering, crush the garlic and let it sit.

Drain the chickpeas. The boiling will have removed a lot of the skins, if you can be bothered, remove these from the sieve before putting the chickpeas into the blender.

Add all the other ingredients (except the water) to the blender and start blending. Add the water little by little while blending until you get a smooth, fluffy consistency.

Enjoy with pitta bread, carrot sticks or salt and pepper crisps mmmm, yummy.

In my opinion, the above recipe makes the best hummus, however, I do appreciate that different people have different tastes, so it is important to taste and adjust according to your palette.

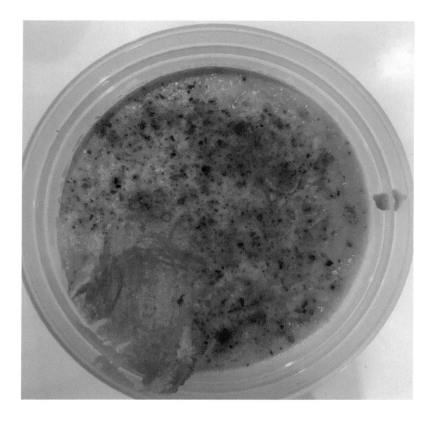

Tapenade

I used to love tapenade so much and would always buy it from the local market, only to find that me and my dad were the only ones who'd eat it. This version is loved by all of my family and doesn't contain anchovies like a normal tapenade. Win win.

Ingredients

180g black olives

170g green olives (nothing fancy is needed, just plain pitted olives)

2 tbsp capers (to replace the tang of the anchovies)

2 tsp miso paste (to give the savouriness of anchovies)

3 tbsp sun dried tomatoes

5 cloves of garlic, crushed

2 tsp mixed herbs

A handful of fresh parsley be sparing, this parsley is vital to the tapenade, however, you can very easily put too much in, so just add a little then taste, then add a little more.

A handful of fresh basil leaves

Juice of ½ a lemon

Glug of extra virgin olive oil to get the right consistency (roughly 60g)

Salt and pepper

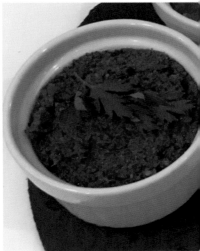

Method

Put all the ingredients into the blender and pulse until you get the consistency that you'd like.

Season to taste and enjoy with fresh ciabatta, oat biscuits or try in 'my take on bruschetta' (pg 146).

Flapjack with an Edge

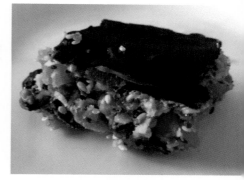

Makes enough for a week to have as a little tea break snack and it is there for any surprise visitors.

You can be a bit creative and if you don't have an ingredient, you can replace it with something similar.

Ingredients

150g pure dairy free spread

120g of local honey

50g coconut oil

A teaspoon of each: cinnamon and mixed spice

½ tsp salt

350g rolled oats

100g of washed and chopped dried apricots

60g of desiccated coconut

50g sesame seeds

50g chia seeds

50g hemp hearts

100g of mixed seeds - pumpkin and sunflower

50g of dried cranberries

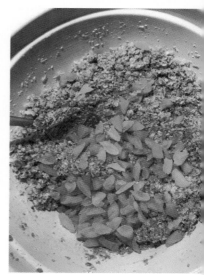

Method

Put the spread, honey and coconut oil into a large microwaveable bowl.

Melt on a low power (350W) in the microwave until all melted.

Stir in the salt, cinnamon and mixed spice.

Stir in the oats until all the oats are coated with the mixture.

Add the chopped fruit and nuts mixture a little at a time, then stir well.

Pour into a clean baking tray and tap down with the back of your spoon to flatten it all down.

I pick out any fruit that is near the edges and drop them into the middle because they tend to catch at the edges.

I cover with tin foil to save anything dropping on to the mixture whilst it's cooking.

Place in the oven 160°C/140°C fan for 30 minutes

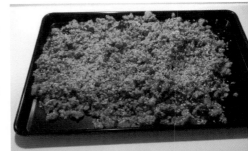

Remove from the oven when it is a light golden brown.

Leave to cool.

For the Chocolate Topping

Melt some chocolate and drizzle over the top, 85% vegan dark chocolate best.

To melt the chocolate, break the chocolate block into bite size pieces and put into a mug. Put in the microwave on a low power (350W).

Once it's melted, drizzle over the top.

Spread the chocolate out with the back of your spoon.

Put the tray into the fridge to set the chocolate, then break it into portion size pieces.

Store in the fridge.

Top tip - Fold the Tin Foil and save for the next time.

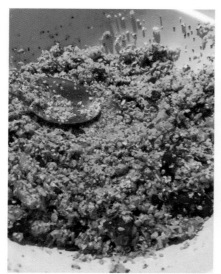

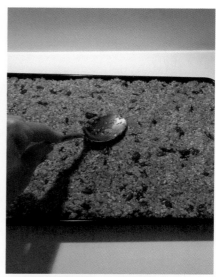

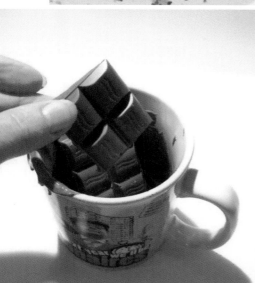

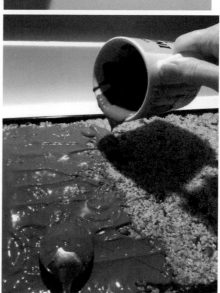

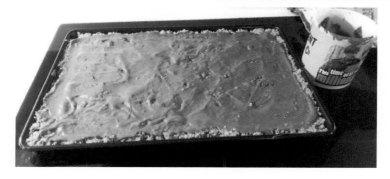

Roasted Chickpeas

An absolutely delicious crunchy, tasty healthy snack or accompaniment to a dish such as baked aubergine.

Ingredients

2 tins of chickpeas

½ tbsp sunflower oil

Generous pinch of salt, pepper, cayenne pepper, paprika and cumin.

Method

Preheat the oven to 200°C/180°C fan.

Drain the tins of chickpeas and rinse thoroughly. Reserve the juice to make some meringues later. Dry the chickpeas on a paper towel or clean tea towel, making sure they are really *really* dry.

Spread the chickpeas out on a non-stick baking tray and bake in a preheated oven for 15 minutes to dry out further.

Remove the tray from the oven and drizzle over the sunflower oil, use a non-metal spoon to stir the chickpeas around to make sure they are all lightly coated in the oil.

Sprinkle on plenty of salt, pepper, cayenne pepper, paprika and cumin (any spicy flavours that you'd like really) and gently stir.

Place the tray back in the oven for another 10 minutes. Stir, then place back in the oven for another 10 - 15 minutes. In total they want to be cooked for about 40 minutes.

Open the oven door a crack to let then cool down and crispen up even more.

Store at room temperature. Eat within 4 days, although in our house they get eaten that day.

Toasties

Makes 1

Ingredients

2 slices of your favourite bread

Non-dairy butter

2 slices of Violife cheese slices

1 large tomato, sliced

2 slices of Quorn Smoky Ham (or any other vegan hams you'd like)

Salt and pepper

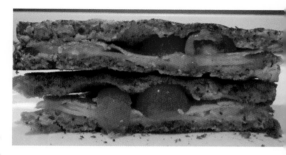

Method

Butter one side of each slice of bread (these will go on the outside of the toastie to ensure crusty bread)

Layer one of the slices with cheese, ham then tomato (the order is important to ensure the cheese doesn't get soggy from the tomatoes)

Season generously with salt and pepper

Place in a preheated toastie machine or onto a hot frying pan for 4-5 minutes and I guarantee that the finished product is comparable to a non-vegan toastie (flip halfway if using a frying pan).

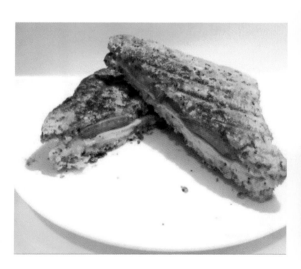
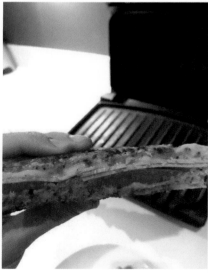

Nutty Banana Bread
Makes 1 loaf

This banana bread is so delicious freshly baked, but also just as delicious a few days old, toasted with butter. Top tip: double the recipe, slice one of the loaves and freeze the slices so when you want a quick snack you can just pop a slice in the toaster, ready to be enjoyed.

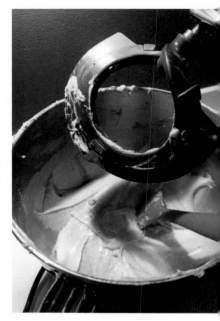

Ingredients

2 flax 'eggs'

115g vegan butter

115g caster sugar

230g self-raising flour (I used gluten free so that my mum could enjoy it, but either work)

1 tsp baking powder (check that it is gluten free if you are intolerant)

1 ripe (ideally brown) banana, roughly mushed

60g walnuts, broken up into smaller pieces **OPTIONAL**

115g sultanas **OPTIONAL**

If nuts and dried fruit aren't your thing, go wild and put some dark chocolate chips in or something, I'm not going to stop you.

Method

Preheat the oven to 200°C/180°C fan.

Make the flax eggs by blending 2 tbsp of flax seeds into a fine powder and mixing with 6 tbsp water, then leaving to sit for 10-15 minutes in the fridge.

While the flax egg is resting, cream together the butter and sugar, either with a wooden spoon or in an electric mixer. The mix should become pale and fluffy.

Then add in your flax eggs and mix well.

Add in the flour and baking powder and mix until the flour is thoroughly incorporated.

Then add in your nuts, sultanas and banana and gently stir by hand.

I do this so that there are nice bits of the bread which are more banana-y, however, if you'd prefer for it to be thoroughly incorporated, mix a bit more vigorously.

Pour into a lined loaf tin (roughly 21 x 11 x 5cm) and put in the oven for 40-50 minutes, or until a skewer poked into it comes out clean.

Take it out of the tin and place onto a wire rack to allow it to cool, then slice and enjoy.

Tips:
- Don't open the oven door halfway through, it is tempting, but the cold air will make the bread lose its rise.
- Err on the side of overcooked rather than undercooked because if it isn't fully baked it will sink, resulting in quite a dense (but still delicious) banana bread.

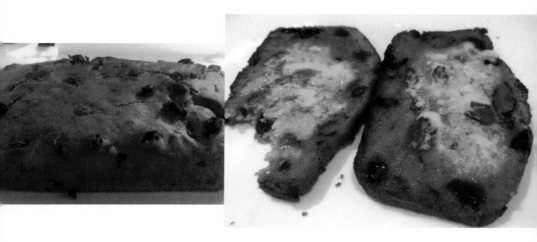

SWEETS - *You will not be able to believe that these are totally plant based. Say no more…*

Grandad Pete's Lemon Drizzle Cake

When I moved into my 2nd year house at university, our new next door neighbours knocked on our door and had brought round some freshly baked lemon drizzle cake (still warm!!!!!), so lemon drizzle cake will always have a special place in my heart.

Ingredients

<u>For the Cake</u>

2 tablespoons of flax seeds

115g of vegan butter, I like to use 'dairy free pure (perfect for baking)' as they use sustainable palm oil

170g caster sugar

4 tablespoons dairy free milk we like to use Alpro oat, but it's your choice

170g of self-raising flour (if you want it gluten free, try to use a good quality flour such as Doves Farm because that makes a big difference)

1 teaspoon of baking powder (if you are gf, make sure you check that your baking powder doesn't have flour in because the cheaper brands sometimes use it to bulk it out/stabilise it)

Zest of 2 lemons (put them to one side after zesting so that they can be used to make the icing)

<u>For the Icing</u>

Juice of 2 lemons

80g of caster sugar

Method

Blitz the flax seeds into a fine powder using a blender or a pestle and mortar (if you don't have either, try to find finely milled flaxseeds, it will result in a slightly grittier cake but it is still nice).

Mix the flax seeds with 6 tablespoons of water and leave in the fridge for 15 minutes until it forms an egg consistency. While the 'egg' is forming, preheat the oven to 190°C/170°C fan and beat the sugar and butter together until pale and creamy.

Add the milk and eggs and mix thoroughly. Sift in the self-raising flour and baking powder, add the lemon zest and stir until it is all combined.

Pour into a large loaf tin and bake for 40 minutes to 1 hour until the outside is golden brown and a skewer comes out clean (while the cake is in the oven, mix the icing together in a jug).

While the cake is hot out of the oven, make a few holes in the top using a skewer or a fork and spoon the icing over, little by little, allowing it to absorb.

Once the cake has cooled, take out of the tin and enjoy (or enjoy it while warm if you can't wait)!

Chocolate Crispy Cakes

Mmmmm I actually love chocolate crispy cakes, they are so easy and so delicious and a perfect little snack for when you want something crunchy.

Ingredients

2 tbsp vegan butter

2 tbsp golden syrup

2 tbsp caster sugar

40g dark chocolate

2 tbsp cocoa powder

2 cups corn flakes/rice krispies (gf if necessary)

NEED: cupcake/muffin cases

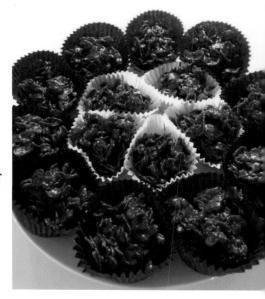

Method

Put the butter, syrup and sugar into a large bowl and microwave on a medium power for about a minute, or until just melted.

Then, stir in the dark chocolate and cocoa powder (the dark chocolate should be melted by the heat of the butter mixture).

Add the corn flakes/rice krispies, little by little, stirring gently so as not to break the cereal, until there is little/no chocolate sauce at the bottom of the bowl.

Spoon into cupcake/muffin cases and refrigerate until firm (or just enjoy while still warm!).

Top tip: if you are using rice krispies, they will go soft if your chocolate mix is too hot so check that it is cool enough for you to dip your finger in before combining.

Seb's Macarons

We love making these macarons because they are naturally gluten free, so my mum can have them, but also it is a fun thing for me and my brothers to make together as it is a real labour of love.

Ingredients

1 400g tin of chickpeas in water, vigorously shaken

¼ tsp of white vinegar

1 small pinch of xanthan gum
OPTIONAL

Pinch of salt

1 tsp vanilla extract

80g caster sugar

100g icing sugar

110g ground almonds

For the Filling

60g vegan butter

25g icing sugar

Favourite jam

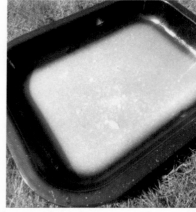

Method

Drain the liquid out of the tin of chickpeas and pour into a pan. (Save the chickpeas for another recipe, for example- hummus (pg 156)).

Bring the chickpea water (aka aquafaba) to a gentle simmer and reduce until it has halved (should weigh roughly 80g at the end).

Pour the aquafaba into a tray and place in the fridge to cool down.

While the aquafaba is cooling, thoroughly wash all whisking utensils, including the bowl as they need to be spotlessly clean to ensure the aquafaba whisks up.

When the aquafaba has cooled to room temp or below, pour into your mixing bowl with the white vinegar, salt and xanthan gum.

Whisk on a high speed until frothy then add the caster sugar, 1 tbsp at a time, ensuring that the sugar is fully mixed in before adding the next tablespoon.

At this point, the mixture should be thick and glossy. Add the vanilla extract and whisk again for a minute until it is mixed in and you have stiff peaks.

You should be able to confidently hold the bowl above your head without worrying that the meringue will come out.

Blend the icing sugar and the ground almonds in a food processor to ensure that they are completely fine and then sift into a bowl.

Fold the sugar and almond mix into the meringue, ⅓rd at a time, making figure eights with your spatula. By now you should have a mixture that flows but isn't too runny. If it is still too thick, keep folding for a bit longer.

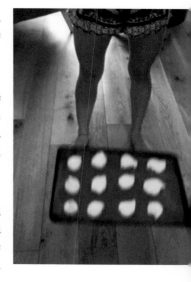

Place a piping bag (or even just a spare sandwich bag) into a long jug and fold the top over the rim of the jug. Spoon the macaron mixture into the piping bag then cut the end off so that you can pipe.

Pipe the macaron mix onto little circles, around 3cm big, on a silicone mat lined baking tray.

Now you have to slam your baking tray on the work surface/drop it on the floor to burst any air bubbles in your mixture, I would advise you to warn

your housemates before you do this. Please ignore how wonky the macarons in the above picture are, we ran out of piping bags and it turns out a bread loaf bag is not a good substitute.

You can now use a toothpick to burst any little bubbles that you can see on the surface-be gentle.

Leave the macarons on the side in your kitchen for a few hours so that they can dry out, before heating the oven to 110°C/100°C fan. Cook the macarons for 25-30 minutes, depending on how big your macarons are.

After that time is up, leave them in the oven for 15 minutes to cool, then prop the door open with a spoon and cool for a further 10 minutes.

Then take the macarons out of the oven and leave to cool on the side.

During this time, you can beat together the ingredients for the filling, adding a little jam at a time, to taste. Alternatively, you can choose a different filling entirely, it's fun to experiment and see what works. We made a lemon curd filling (pg 169) which was delicious, however, caused our macarons to disintegrate overnight.

Assemble and enjoy.

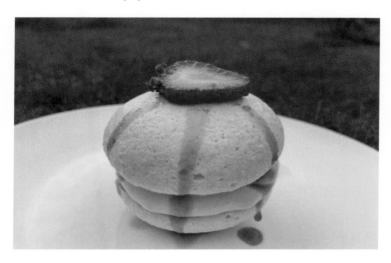

Dorset Apple Cake

This is sooo delicious, I literally made one this morning and it's all gone already. Now I want to bake another one.

It's not very traditional, it is kind of a crossover between an apple upside down cake and a Dorset apple cake. Using cooking apples means that they sort of disintegrate into a delicious, tangy (because of the lemon) jam and the actual cake is caramel-y and chewy and just ridiculously tasty.

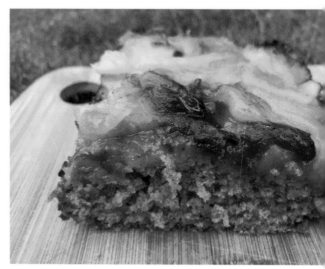

Ingredients

1 flax 'egg'

1½ large cooking apples, peeled, cored and cut into angel wings

1 tbsp lemon juice (half a lemon)

1 tsp baking powder (add ½ tsp more baking powder with 1 tsp milk if you're making gf)

110g plain flour (gf works)

100g caster sugar

Pinch of salt

1 tsp cinnamon

1 tsp vanilla extract

75g vegan butter, melted

Sprinkle of dark brown sugar

Method

Preheat the oven to 200°C/180°C fan.

Make the flax egg by blending 1 tbsp flax seeds into a fine powder. Mix the flax seed powder with 3 tbsp of water and let set in the fridge for 15 minutes.

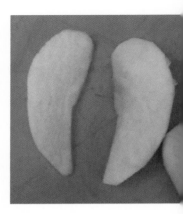

Prepare the apples and drizzle with lemon juice to keep fresh.

Put the flour, baking powder, sugar, salt and cinnamon into a bowl and start beating.

Gradually add the melted butter, vanilla extract and the eggs until well mixed.

Grease a 21 x 11 x 6cm loaf tin and layer the apple slices in the bottom. Sprinkle over the dark brown sugar and then add the cake mix.

Bake for 40-50 minutes, you don't have to worry about overcooking it, because you want a nice chewy exterior to counteract the sweet and tangy apple base.

Leave to cool in the tin for 10 minutes then turn out onto a wire rack to cool.

Enjoy with some vegan single cream.

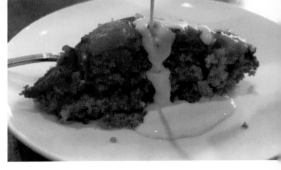

Peppermint Chocolate Heart
Serves 6

Ingredients

180g dark chocolate (or 1 bar of chocolate)
12 drops of organic peppermint oil

A sprinkling of icing sugar, a mint leaf and
a raspberry to decorate.

In the picture to the right we served it with
half a vegan truffle!

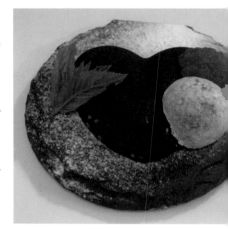

Method

Break the chocolate up into a microwaveable mug.

Very gently heat in the microwave on a low power until the chocolate has
melted - roughly 4 minutes, stirring occasionally.

Add the drops of organic peppermint essential oil.

Pour into a heart shaped mould.

Put in the fridge to cool, if you want it to stay shiny, let it cool at room
temperature.

Turn out and serve, it's just simple and yummy.

**If peppermint isn't your thing, feel free to use orange extract, vanilla
extract, almond extract, whatever you fancy. You can also add a little
more sugar to make it sweeter if you'd like. Flavoured vegan
chocolate is often expensive/ difficult to get hold of so just flavouring
your own dark chocolate is a perfect way to subdue those chocolate
cravings.**

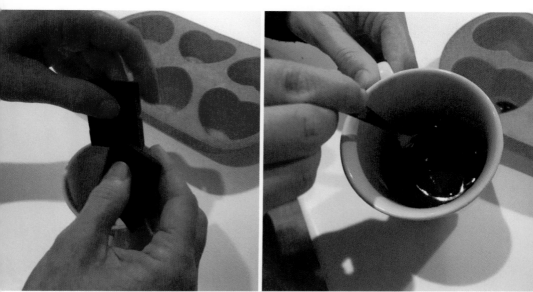

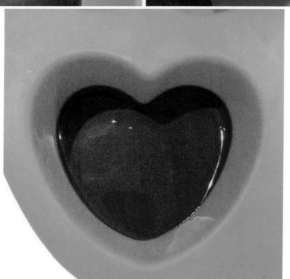

Coconut Chia Pudding

Serves 6

Ingredients

80g chia seeds

600ml coconut milk (1 and a half tins)

1 tsp vanilla extract

Pinch of salt

Serve with

Fresh berries

Raspberry coulis (pg 121)

Method

Whisk all the ingredients together and pour into 6 glass bowls.

Leave to set in the fridge for a few hours.

Enjoy with fresh berries and raspberry coulis.

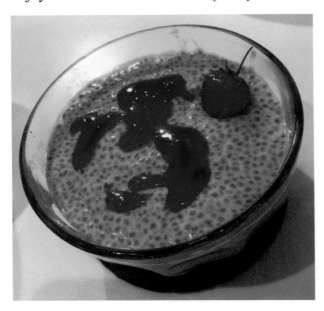

Gluten Free Brownie

This recipe is inspired by a gluten free brownie recipe off BBC GoodFood and it is by far the best gluten free one that I've tried, I honestly think you can't tell that it contains no gluten, or animal products! It turns out less like a bakery brownie and more like the sort of brownie you'd get at a restaurant, not very chewy, but very rich and airy. It is best enjoyed with a drizzle of vegan single cream, or some vegan vanilla ice cream. If you're not gluten intolerant, just make with ordinary plain flour.

Ingredients

4 flax eggs

250g vegan butter

250g dark chocolate

300g caster sugar

1 tsp vanilla extract

100g gluten free plain flour

60g cocoa powder

1 tsp salt

Optional Extras

175g vegan chocolate chips

200g fresh cherries, pitted

175g raisins

Whatever you fancy, go for it

Method

Preheat the oven to 180°C/160°C fan.

Make the flax eggs by blending 4 tbsp flax seeds into fine pieces, mixing with 12 tbsp water and letting sit for 15 minutes in the fridge.

Melt the vegan butter in the microwave on a low heat then add the chocolate and stir in until melted.

Whisk the flax eggs with the sugar for a few minutes then mix in the melted butter and chocolate, vanilla extract, flour, cocoa powder and salt. Beat until incorporated then add in any extras you'd like.

Pour the brownie mix into a lined baking tray (BBC GoodFood recommends 30x20cm, however, if you'd prefer a thicker brownie, pour it into a shorter baking tray) and bake for 30-35 minutes.

Leave to cool completely in the tin, or tuck in while it's still warm if you just can't resist.

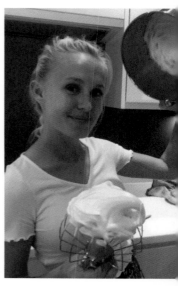

Raspberry Pavlova

Ingredients

1 400g tin of chickpeas, vigorously shaken (so that the water contains all the sediment from the chickpeas)

¼ tsp white vinegar

1 tsp vanilla extract

¼ tsp xanthan gum

105g caster sugar (granulated won't work)

45g icing sugar

1 tin of full fat coconut milk, refrigerated to help the cream separate (or you could use a shop bought vegan double cream)

200g raspberry jam (or whatever your favourite jam is)

Raspberry coulis (pg 121)

Handful of raspberries and blueberries

Method

Drain the chickpea water into a saucepan and set aside the chickpeas for another recipe (for example the falafel salad on pg 44).

Simmer the chickpea water (aka aquafaba) on the stove until it has halved in volume (it should weigh around 80g after it has reduced).

Once the aquafaba has halved, spread it out on a small tray to allow it to cool (you can put it in the fridge if you'd like to speed up the cooling).

Preheat the oven to 120°C/100°C fan.

When the aquafaba is at room temperature, pour into a mixing bowl with the vinegar, vanilla extract and xanthan gum and whisk on a high speed until it starts to get frothy.

It is imperative that your mixing bowl and whisk are spotless, so wash it before use. My mum used to always swear by swiping a lemon half around the bowl but I'm not sure if that really makes any difference.

While the mixer is running, add the caster sugar 1 tbsp at a time, waiting after each time to ensure that the sugar has dissolved fully.

Continue adding caster sugar and whisking until the meringue has formed stiff peaks. This means that you can hold it over your head without it moving.

Now sift in the icing sugar, and gently fold it into the meringue with a spatula, 15g at a time.

How to fold: gently make a figure eight motion through your mixture, turning the bowl as you go until everything is incorporated. You must be careful to not knock the air out of the mixture or you will end up with a deflated meringue.

Spoon the meringue onto a lined baking tray into whatever shape you fancy, however, I did round with a dent in the middle for the cream. Bake for 2 hours.

Silicon mats work best for lining the baking tray, but I wouldn't worry too much if you're just using greaseproof paper.

After the 2 hours are up, turn the oven off but DO NOT OPEN THE DOOR. It is very important that the meringue cools down gradually so that it doesn't collapse. This takes a minimum of 3 hours, but ideally overnight.

Store in an airtight container until you are ready to serve (as toppings will cause the meringue to collapse if done too long in advance). When you are ready to serve, spoon the firm white part of the coconut milk (the cream) into a mixing bowl, add the raspberry jam and whisk until light and fluffy.

You can add more/less raspberry jam depending on your personal taste.

Spoon the coconut cream into the centre of the meringue and garnish with fresh fruit, raspberry coulis and icing sugar. Enjoy ASAP.

These toppings are just guidance, if you're more of a nutty person, mix some cocoa powder/vegan Nutella into the cream and serve with hazelnuts on top, or go bananas and serve with caramel and bananas. The world of pavlovas is your oyster.

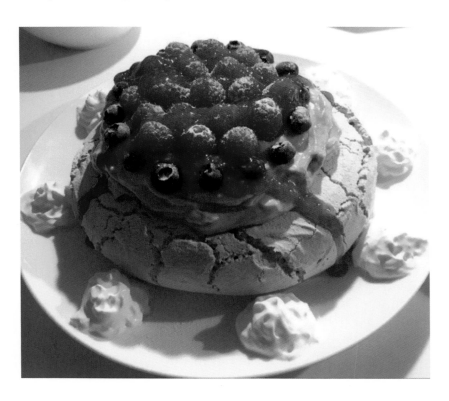

Banoffee Pie

My oh my, I cannot tell you how good this banoffee pie is. Admittedly, it has always been my favourite dessert, but this version really takes the biscuit (pun intended). I made it for my boyfriend's non-vegan family and they said it's better than an ordinary one. Don't worry about being able to taste coconut, when it is all together, it isn't noticeable, but if you're concerned, feel free to adjust the amount of vanilla extract added to the caramel, to your taste.

Ingredients

Base

225g of plain vegan biscuits, crushed into a fine crumb (I used Hobnobs, however, they contain palm oil so if you can find a vegan biscuit with sustainably sourced palm oil/none at all, please let me know)

150g of vegan butter (you want a butter that is fairly hard when refrigerated because that will help to make a sturdy base, if you can't find a good vegan butter, coconut oil will work as it is solid at room temp, however, it will result in a fairly coconutty base)

Caramel

330g brown sugar (it's important that it is brown as it will give it a more caramel colour)

2 tins of <u>full fat</u> coconut milk, which have been stored upright in the fridge to ensure that the cream is separate (I got Blue Dragon for this, it is well worth the extra money because you want the thick cream part of the tin, not the liquid at the bottom, and cheaper coconut milk has far less cream)

2 tbsp vanilla extract

1 tsp salt

Caramelised banana **OPTIONAL**

1 banana

30g caster sugar

1 tbsp hot water

Knob of vegan butter

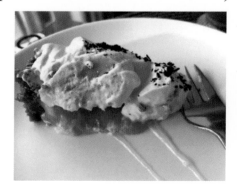

To serve

1 banana

270ml vegan double cream (I like Elmea best, if you can't find any, use another tin of coconut milk, take the cream off the top and whip with icing sugar until it is like whipped cream)

Block of dark chocolate to grate on top

Method

Crush the biscuits with a food processor or rolling pin while melting the butter (I prefer to melt it in the microwave on a lower power setting, but if you prefer to do it over a bain-marie or in a pan, do your thing).

Pour the melted butter in with the biscuits and stir to combine. Pour the buttery biscuit crumbs into a 20cm diameter tin, ideally with a removable bottom and press into the base and up the sides to form a buttery biscuit base (see the picture). I used my thumbs and knuckles to press the biscuits into the desired shape, but the back of a spoon would work too.

Place the base in the fridge for at least an hour to set, you want it to be nice and firm so that it can hold the banoffee pie together.

Now it's time to get cracking with the caramel. Do not be afraid, it is extremely easy. Heat a saucepan on the hob on a medium-high heat and pour in the brown sugar, stirring occasionally until it has heated through (around 2 mins).

Now you want to add in the coconut cream, salt and vanilla extract. This means opening your tin of coconut milk, scooping out the firm white bit and adding it to the sugar. Try to get as little coconut water in as possible as that can cause crystallisation. Don't worry if you don't scrape all the coconut cream out, just get as much as you can with a spoon.

Stir to combine and bring to the boil, then simmer for around 15-20 minutes. Don't stir too regularly as this will slow down the process.

It will thicken as it cools, so a good way to check if it is done is to spread a tsp of the caramel onto a plate and refrigerate it for a few minutes then check the consistency.

If it is the right consistency, remove it from the heat and allow it to cool for a little while (20 minutes) at room temp, before pouring it into the biscuit base to set for 1 hour in the fridge.

While the caramel sets in the base, slice one of the bananas in diagonal slices and prepare to make some caramelised banana **OPTIONAL**.

Heat the sugar and water in a frying pan, on a medium high heat until it forms a caramel. Add the diagonal banana slices and swirl around, allowing the caramel to coat them.

Add the knob of butter to the pan and cook for a few minutes then transfer the banana slices to a plate.

Whip up your vegan double cream of choice into stiff peaks and slice the remaining banana in diagonal slices.

If the caramel and the biscuit base are cold and set it is assembly time. Lay the caramelised bananas on top of the caramel, then spoon on the whipped cream. After that, layer on the fresh bananas and finally, garnish with a grating of dark chocolate. Enjoy.

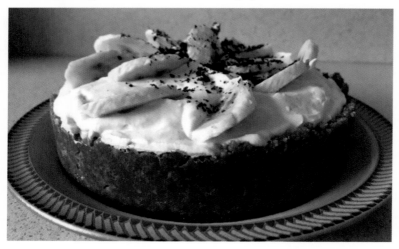

Sorbets

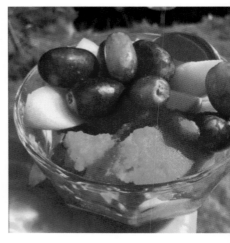

Vegan sorbets are -

* incredibly easy to make
* super refreshing on a hot day and
* a great way to save fruit that needs eating up

Warning, you do need a fairly strong blender as you will be blending frozen fruit, you could try letting it defrost a little and then blending, and adding less water, however a good blender is well worth the investment if you want to eat more plant-based.

The key thing to remember is the ratio

20:7:5   fruit:water:sugar

So if you have 20g of fruit, mix in 7ml of water and 5g of sugar

Or, if you have 200g of fruit, you mix in 70ml of water and 50g of sugar (just multiply by 10)

Or, if you have 60g of fruit, mix in 21ml of water and 15g sugar

Method

Cut up whatever fruit you'd like and weigh how much you have - remember this number - then pop it into a Tupperware pot and into the freezer for around 2 hours, I find that if you freeze it for longer than 2 hours, it sometimes gets so cold that you can't taste the fruit as much, so if you do it overnight, leave the fruit on the side for a little while to defrost slightly.

Use that number to calculate how much water and sugar you will need, using the ratio above.

Then, add the sugar to the water in a jug and heat up in the microwave until the sugar has dissolved. Leave this for a few hours as well (but in the fridge), to allow it to cool.

~A few hours later~

Put the frozen fruit into a blender and blend, adding the sugar water little by little, until you have a nice, smooth sorbet consistency.

If you have the patience, you can actually put this sorbet back into the freezer (still in the blender) then bring it out an hour or 2 later and blend again. This makes the sorbet unbelievably creamy and I would recommend, but it does require a very strong blender.

Serve with some fresh fruit and enjoy…

Our favourite sorbet flavours are -

- Pear
- Mango
- Pineapple
- Kiwi
- Melon (as this is quite a sweet fruit, try making with less sugar or you risk it being a little sickly)
- Watermelon (as this has a high water content, you may not need to add in all the water)

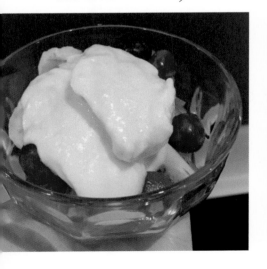
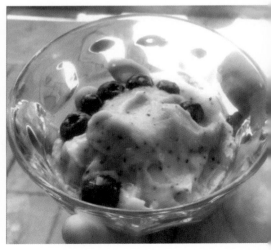

Easy Ice Cream

Serves 6

Method

Chop 4 *very ripe* bananas into small pieces and put in the freezer for a few hours (or overnight).

If your bananas aren't very ripe, it will still work, it just won't be as sweet so you might want to add some sugar/maple syrup when you're blending.

Put the frozen pieces in a blender and blend until smooth.

Adding some plant milk (around 1 tbsp) can help to get a nice creamy consistency.

It will go into some weird frozen chunks at first, just have patience, scrape down the sides if you need to, and keep blending because it will go really creamy.

Flavour Ideas

- Roast 200g of hazelnuts at 180°C for 10-12 minutes. After they are done, roll them around on the tray/in your hands to get the skins off. Blend with ¼ tsp of salt until it becomes buttery. Add that to the banana ice cream with some cocoa powder for a Nutella flavour ice cream.

- Add 1½ tbsp of vanilla extract for vanilla ice cream.

- Add 2tsp of peppermint and 100g of dark chocolate chips for mint-choc-chip.

- Make your own vegan caramel (pg 181) and make banoffee pie flavoured ice cream.

The world is your oyster, have a fun time and experiment.

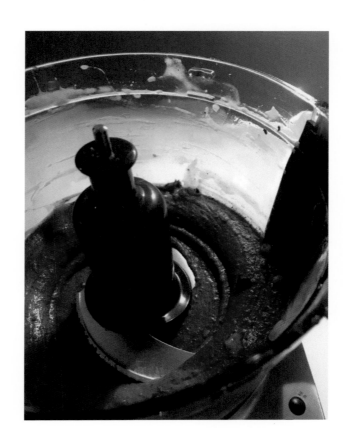

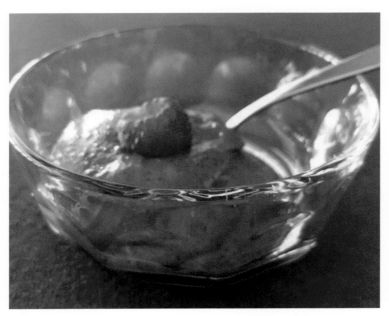

Equipment

This a comprehensive list of the kitchen equipment we regularly use.

Large Pyrex microwaveable bowl.

Pyrex jug for peas, sauces etc.

Pyrex bowl with edges so that you can pick it up if it's hot.

Microwavable bowl with a handle for cooking porridge in the morning, to save on washing up, have it the size so that you can make it without it boiling over, cook it and eat out of it ... boom!

One large frying pan with a lid.

One large stainless-steel lid pan for boiling pasta, rice, noodles etc.

Pie dish 30 x 28 x 8 cm.

Casserole dish 38 x 26 x 6cm.

3 baking trays (26 x 38 x 2cm) or whatever fits in your oven.

Cake tin, 20 cm diameter x 4cm deep.

Loaf tin 21 x 11 x 5.

Food processor if you can afford one	Mug
Hand/ stick blender	Can opener
Hand balloon whisk and potato masher	Of course, a chopping board and a sharp knife
Sieve/colander	Silicone reusable baking parchment.
Measuring spoon (tsp and tbsp)	Muffin cases
Silicon spatula	Electric mixer for baking

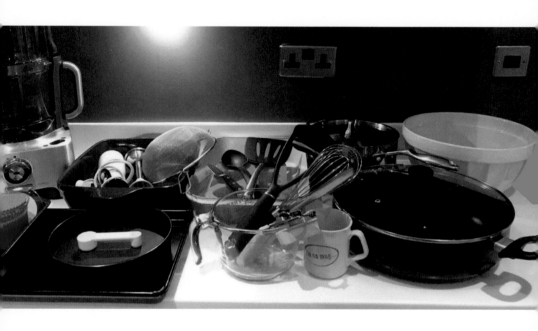

Index

Apple, 172
Aubergine, 61, 118, 120, 154, 162
Avocado, 18, 98, 147
Banana, 34, 164, 181, 186, 191
Berries, 34, 176
Broccoli, 56, 86, 88, 94, 125
Butternut Squash, 76, 100
Cabbage, 40, 41, 78, 94, 135
Carrot, 52, 97, 145, 157
Cashew, 56, 58, 66, 84, 86, 89, 110, 112, 134, 138
Cauliflower, 19, 155
Celery, 47, 78, 79, 105
Chocolate, 121, 160, 164, 168, 174, 177, 178, 182, 186
Mango, 40, 185
Mushrooms, 38, 50, 66, 72, 74, 76, 78, 81, 84, 88, 102, 105, 110, 114, 120, 132, 134
Peas, 48, 50, 55, 56, 61, 66, 79, 84, 85, 102, 104, 105, 135, 148
Pineapple, 35, 132, 134
Potato, 41, 71, 118
Sausage, 38, 64
Spinach, 56, 58, 64, 101, 108, 111, 118, 142, 145
Sweet Potato, 48, 73, 76, 91, 98, 108, 140
Sweetcorn, 48, 55, 84, 96, 105, 108, 132

Definitions of Unfamiliar Ingredients

Here I have listed any ingredients used in my book which may be unfamiliar or unusual. Although they may seem intimidating, all of these can be bought easily at most big supermarkets in the UK.

Aquafaba: The water from a tin of chickpeas (aka aquafaba), is extremely high in protein from the chickpeas, so works just like egg whites. It is perfect for making meringues and mousses and other funky animal-based desserts. It also reduces waste which is obviously a bonus.

Bamboo Shoots: Most often found tinned in supermarkets, bamboo shoots are just young bamboo plants. They are often found in Chinese cuisine and have a very tasty, refreshing flavour. They are high in potassium and other vitamins and minerals.

Banana Blossom: Literally the blossom of the banana, it is already widely eaten in South-East Asia, but is starting to become popular in vegan cuisine as it has a very meaty/ fishy texture and mild taste. Can be found tinned in Sainsburys.

Chia Seeds: Tiny seeds which actually come from a plant in the mint family, chia seeds are very high in fibre, omega-3, protein and calcium (more than milk). They also are shown to help improve satiety, so they are a good thing to sprinkle over your breakfast to help keep you going until lunch.

Edamame Beans: Immature soybeans, still in their pods, edamame beans have a mild, nutty flavour so are perfect as a side with a curry. They have all the same benefits as the other soy products on this list, high in protein, lower cholesterol, reduce risk of certain types of cancer, the list goes on. Some people are concerned about soy interfering with thyroid function; however, most studies show that as long as your diet contains iodine, there is nothing to worry about.

Flax Seeds: Technically a superfood, flax seeds are high in protein, omega-3, fibre, help to control blood sugar and may be shown to reduce blood pressure. The handiest thing about flax seeds though, is that they absorb water, giving them a gloopy, egg-like consistency.

Hemp: Hemp is essentially an all-round amazing plant, I can't write enough here about it, but if you go to https://www.goodhemp.com you can find out all about it yourself. The main summary is that hemp plants absorb 4x more CO_2 than trees; they need no pesticides; and growing them actually replenishes the soil they're in. Not just that, the plants grow hemp hearts which are supposedly the best source of plant based protein on the planet, they are uber high in fibre and good fats *and* they can be grown in France, meaning few air miles. Hemp hearts are classed as a superfood, but they are also very tasty and can be sprinkled on basically anything, to just add an extra bit of protein.

Jackfruit: Similar to banana blossom, jackfruit is not a new invention, it is a fruit that has been grown and eaten in South-East Asia for a long time. It is now becoming used more in vegan cuisine to mimic chicken and it has a very similar texture and absorbs flavours well.

Miso Paste (me-so): A Japanese paste made of fermented soybeans, miso paste is the definition of the flavour umami (basically the taste of savoury-ness). It comes in varying colours; the darker ones have been fermented

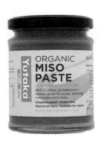 for longer and so have a stronger flavour. As it is fermented, it is good to add into 'cheesy' dishes as it helps mimic the fermented flavour of cheese. It is normally gluten free, however, sometimes other things are added (such as barley or rice) to give a different flavour, so make sure you check the back if you're intolerant.

Mirin: A type of rice wine, similar to sake, but a lot sweeter and less alcoholic.

Nori: Used a lot in Japanese food, nori is edible seaweed, so is very good at bringing a 'taste of the sea' to vegan food in place of fish. Is also used to wrap sushi.

Nutritional Yeast: The same species of yeast as makes beer, but deactivated, and used to give a nutty/cheesy flavour to food. It's most notable health benefit is that it is high in B vitamins, which vegans often struggle to get as they are predominantly found in meat and dairy. Looks a bit like fish food, but dissolves as soon as it's mixed with sauce.

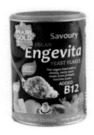

Quinoa (keen-wah): A seed that is often treated as a grain, it is a complete protein, high in fibre, gluten free and classed as a superfood.

Sake (sah-kay): Rice wine, made by fermenting rice, in a similar way to how beer is made. Very common in Japanese cuisine.

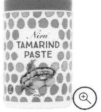

Tamarind: A fruit native to Asia and Africa, it is both sweet and slightly sour at the same time and is used to make Worcester sauce. It is sold as a paste in most supermarkets, but if you can't find it, your closest Asian supermarket will definitely have it.

Tempeh (temp-ay): A block, made from cooked soya beans, which have then been fermented. It is a complete protein, higher in protein than tofu and has a subtle nutty taste. Tempeh must be cooked for 20 minutes minimum, but other than that, can be used interchangeably with tofu.

Tofu (toe-foo): A block made from soya milk that has been condensed down. A good source of protein, lowers bad cholesterol, possibly reduces breast cancer, and helps with menopause symptoms. Comes in two different types: firm and silken, firm can be squeezed and fried/ baked to give a meaty texture, whereas silken is a lot softer and creamier, good for making protein packed sauces. Tofu is what my friend calls "negative flavour" so it works really well in saucy dishes as it absorbs the flavour easily.

Water Chestnuts: A prominent ingredient in Chinese food, water chestnuts are roots that have grown in freshwater and are a good source of potassium, fibre and contain little fat. They have a very mild flavour, but are nice and crunchy, mostly found tinned in supermarkets.

A FINAL WORD

Dad - As a 'typical male' I have spent my life eating, and enjoying, a lot of meat. Like most dad's, I have learned a lot from my kids. I was initially sceptical when Emilia introduced the idea of a plant-based diet to the family. But having watched Game Changers and Cowspiracy I became open to the idea and thought I'd give it a go - with no real intention of it becoming a long-term lifestyle change - what harm could it do? I am also really concerned about the environment and it is clear that the current global population cannot support beef consumption on the current scale.

However, the changes to my life have been profound. Doing a lot of exercise, I have come to accept aching joints and muscle pain as an inevitable part of growing older. I could not have been more wrong. Changing my diet has largely eliminated those pains and I feel that I am fitter and more well than I have been in twenty years. Another major win is that keeping my weight down has always been a challenge. The advantage of this diet is that you can eat what you like, feel full and stay in shape. So, it really has been transformative - give it a go, what have you got to lose?

Mum - Well... my cholesterol was on the high side, I watched Game Changers and I thought 'why not'. I haven't looked back (well after the first week or two). My cholesterol and all my other bloods have come back better than I could have imagined. Added to that, I now actually can't believe that I ever thought that it was okay to kill an animal for me. This is from the girl that used to pluck hundreds of turkeys at Christmas!

Seb - I went vegan, originally for health reasons, however, as I delved deeper into the plant-based lifestyle, I came to realise that you could lead a healthier life (I can run quicker and further than I ever could before) with the added benefit of not causing harm to sentient beings. In addition, being plant based is better for the environment, therefore, I can't really understand why anyone would still eat meat. I think, in the future, we will look back on people eating meat, the same way we look back on gladiators fighting to a barbaric death. It is an ancient practice, which needs to stop.

Theo - I originally only went plant-based because I had moved back in with my family for the holidays, however, after cooking and eating plant-based food for roughly 6 months, I have noticed such a huge impact on my overall fitness. Now, when I go back to uni, I won't be eating meat or dairy. It is significantly cheaper and healthier to eat tins of beans, lentils and the wide expanse of new vegan products than it would be to have a steak. Finally, I love being able to appreciate the world and its wildlife without having subliminal guilt.

Me - I went vegan initially because of environmental impact. I am by no means militant, I will eat cheese if I'm at a friend's house and they have made me dinner, because I don't think that drinking milk is inherently wrong, I just believe that it is unsustainable when there are almost 8 billion people wanting to drink milk too. This unprecedented demand results in bad living quality for the animals and unrealistic pressures on farmers who have to try to keep up for miniscule pay from the big supermarkets. I don't want you to see this cookbook as a strict rulebook, you have to listen to your body, but by eating even one plant based meal each week you are making a positive impact.

I have always loved cooking but going vegan has really enhanced this love. When you start to get the hang of vegan cooking, it is such a joy to create new takes on old favourites and reinvent dishes to be tastier and guilt free. I love walking in the countryside and seeing all the sheep and cows and other animals and now I can enjoy them without the knot in my stomach, knowing that I am responsible for harming them. Also, due to the huge shift in interest, every time I go shopping I swear there are newer and better animal alternatives (and because I am a nerd, I get very excited by this).

Finally, a huge thank you to my wonderful family for helping me actually bring this to life, I couldn't have done it without their help; proofreading, eating my failed attempts, keeping me sane when I'd been working on it all day.

Also, a big thank you to my wonderful friends who have helped me along the way too.

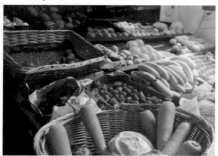
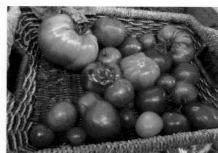

Some photos of the delicious, fresh, plastic-free veg at my local market!

Printed in Great Britain
by Amazon